AF863351

WP
522 A woman's guide to
W872 menopause and hormone
1998 replacement therapy

Health Science Library
St. Joseph's Medical Center
Brainerd, Minnesota

DEMCO

A Woman's Guide to Menopause and Hormone Replacement Therapy

A Woman's Guide to Menopause and Hormone Replacement Therapy

Edited by
Lorraine Dennerstein
and
Julia Shelley

American Psychiatric Press, Inc.

Washington, DC
London, England

Note: The authors have worked to ensure that all information in this book concerning drug dosages, schedules, and routes of administration is accurate as of the time of publication and consistent with standards set by the U.S. Food and Drug Administration and the general medical community. As medical research and practice advance, however, therapeutic standards may change. For this reason and because human and mechanical errors sometimes occur, we recommend that readers follow the advice of a physician who is directly involved in their care or the care of a member of their family.

Books published by the American Psychiatric Press, Inc., represent the views and opinions of the individual authors and do not necessarily represent the policies and opinions of the Press or the American Psychiatric Association.

Copyright © 1998 American Psychiatric Press, Inc.
ALL RIGHTS RESERVED
Manufactured in the United States of America on acid-free paper
01 00 99 98 4 3 2 1
First Edition

American Psychiatric Press, Inc.
1400 K Street, N.W., Washington, DC 20005
www.appi.org

Library of Congress Cataloging-in-Publication Data
A woman's guide to menopause and hormone replacement therapy / edited by Lorraine Dennerstein and Julia Shelley. — 1st ed.
p. cm.
Includes bibliographical references and index.
ISBN 0-88048-782-8 (alk. paper)
1. Menopause—Hormone therapy. 2. Osteoporosis—Hormone therapy. 3. Estrogen—Therapeutic use. 4. Women—Health and hygiene.
I. Dennerstein, Lorraine. II. Shelley, Julia.
[DNLM: 1. Estrogen Replacement Therapy. 2. Menopause—psychology. 3. Osteoporosis, Postmenopausal—prevention & control. 4. Women's Health. WP 522 W872 1998]
RG186.W655 1998
618.1'75—dc21
DNLM/DLC
for Library of Congress 98-10653
CIP

British Library Cataloguing in Publication Data
A CIP record is available from the British Library.

Contents

Contributors

Henry G. Burger, A.O., M.D., M.R.A.C.P., F.R.A.C.P., F.R.A.C.O.G. (Endocrinology); Director, Prince Henry's Institute of Medical Research, Monash Medical Centre, Melbourne, Australia

Jeanne Daly, M.Env.Sc., Ph.D (Sociology)
Senior Lecturer, School of Public Health, La Trobe University, Melbourne, Australia

Lorraine Dennerstein, A.O., M.B.B.S., Ph.D., D.P.M., F.R.A.N.Z.C.P. (Psychiatry); Director, Office for Gender and Health, Department of Psychiatry, The University of Melbourne, Melbourne, Australia

Janet Guthrie, M.Sc., Dip.Ed.(Tert) (Physiology); Research Officer, Office for Gender and Health, Department of Psychiatry, The University of Melbourne, Melbourne, Australia

Assunta Hunter, B.A.(Hons)Soc., N.D. (Naturopathy); Lecturer in Herbal Medicine, Southern School of Natural Therapies, Melbourne, Australia

Malkah T. Notman, M.D. (Psychiatry); Clinical Professor of Psychiatry, Harvard Medical School, and Director of Faculty Development, The Cambridge Hospital, Cambridge, Massachusetts, U.S.A.

Diane Palmer, M.B.B.S., F.R.A.C.O.G. (Gynecology); Gynaecologist, Menopause Clinic, Monash Medical Centre, Melbourne, Australia

Julia Shelley, M.P.H., Ph.D. (Epidemiology); Senior Research Fellow, Centre for the Study of Mothers' and Children's Health, La Trobe University, Melbourne, Australia

Ann Westmore, B.Sc., M.Sc., Journalism (Specialist Health and Science Writer), Melbourne, Australia

Preface

Whether women should or should not take hormone replacement therapy (HRT) remains a hotly contested issue. This book arose to meet women's requests for balanced information that they could view confidently, where several sides of this complex issue could be aired in the one publication.

We offer the reader the opinions of a number of experts from various disciplinary backgrounds. The authors drew on their own and others' published research, including population-based studies, which provide a sense of what most women will experience during the midlife transition, as well as intervention studies. Most studies published to date were carried out in the United States, Europe, and Australia, and few of these involved women from ethnic minority groups. There likewise have been few studies of menopause from the developing world.

Each of the chapters represents the author's own views and biases, as indeed do all opinions. We have not sought to remove overlap or contradiction between the chapters, because the similarities and differences between viewpoints are an important aspect of debate around an issue that is both complex and surrounded by much scientific uncertainty. Indeed, we encourage our readers to bear in mind that this debate is far from over and that further research and discussion will continue to contribute to our understanding of the role of HRT in midlife and beyond.

This book embraces the Principles of Good Practice relevant to Women's Health, developed as a global project by the Commonwealth Secretariat, an intergovernmental body based in London. Health is defined positively according to these principles, and its different dimensions are recognized. The life-cycle perspective of health is taken. The authors recognize the importance of a wide range of determinants of women's health experiences, especially social factors. The diversity of women's experiences are acknowledged by the authors, although there is limited documentation of these at present. The book authorship is multidisciplinary. The book arose from suggestions made by a Community Advisory Committee and sets out to address questions asked of field workers by midlife women. The authors have sought to pass knowledge gained from research directly to women themselves.

The energy and input of a number of people have contributed to the production of this book. We would particularly like to thank Liz River and Kym Clifford, of the Office for Gender and Health, and Carol Nadelson, M.D., Editor-in-Chief of the American Psychiatric Press, for their assistance with the production of the book. We are also indebted to the many women who have participated in our research. Even where we are not drawing directly on research results, input from women in the community is vital for the development of the ideas and views such as those found in this book.

Last, we would like to express our appreciation to the funders of the Melbourne Women's Midlife Health Project.[1]

Julia Shelley
Lorraine Dennerstein

[1]The Melbourne Women's Midlife Health Project has received its major funding from the Victorian Health Promotion Foundation and the Public Health and Research Development Committee of the National Health and Medical Research Council. Grants in aid have also been received from the Australian Dairy Corporation and the following charitable trusts: Percy Baxter Trust, H. and L. Hecht Trust, Estate of the late Daniel Scott, Ian Potter Foundation, Smorgon Family Trust, Leigh and Marjorie Bronwen Murray Charitable Trust, ANZ Trustees, and the Helen Schutt Trust.

Abbreviations

DES: diethylstilbestrol
DXA: dual-energy X-ray absorptiometry
FSH: follicle-stimulating hormone
HDL: high-density lipoprotein
HRT: hormone replacement therapy
LDL: low-density lipoprotein
LH: luteinizing hormone
PEPI: Postmenopausal Estrogen/Progestin Interventions [Trial]
SERM: selective estrogen receptor modulator
WHO: World Health Organization

CHAPTER 1

Hormone Replacement Therapy: The Question for Midlife

Jeanne Daly

To HRT or not to HRT?

The midlife woman is in some ways similar to Hamlet. In Shakespeare's play, Hamlet debates whether "to be or not to be." This is a simple question, but before Hamlet finds his answer (and ceases to be), he has to undergo various trials, which he describes in telling dialogue and moving speeches.

The answer to Hamlet's question is complex and multifaceted. Some women face similar, if less serious, dilemmas as they negotiate midlife. They, too, may see no simple answer. Certainly, the belief that their problems will be solved by a doctor's prescription for hormone replacement therapy (HRT) is too simple an answer.

This chapter shows why this should be so, drawing on the results of interviews with 150 women conducted as part of the La Trobe University study of women's experience of menopause.[1] These results are not reported in detail here but have been used to illustrate the dilemma faced by women in midlife.

How do women see the menopause? First of all, it should be borne in mind that women are accustomed to hormonal fluctuations in each menstrual cycle and during pregnancy. They know what these hormonal changes feel like and have learned to associate certain "ups and downs" with these fluctuations. Menopause is a disruption of their usual patterns. It can take the form of unusually irregular periods, heavy bleeding, or increasing premenstrual stress. On the other hand, some women say that they do not have one or more readily identifiable problems but rather that they feel as though their bodies have gone out of balance. Their brains feel blocked, their digestion starts malfunctioning, their limbs ache, and their bodies can no longer regulate temperature. Some women feel hot all the time, and some have tremendous flashes of heat that leave them dripping wet. Others feel hot inside but cold outside. Women may have these problems one at a time or all together, and in some the problems vary from week to week in both nature and intensity.

This variation is important for two reasons. First, it means that women may see themselves as menopausal long before their periods stop. The medical literature refers to the stage when changes start happening as the *perimenopause* and uses the term *menopause* to describe the actual cessation of menstruation. Women, however, commonly see the cessation of menstruation as one mark along a series of experiences that they associate with the menopause. Second, menopause involves a considerable variety of experiences. If women were mapped along a spectrum, at one end there would be the relatively small number who have serious difficulties in

---

[1] The La Trobe University study, "The Social Construction of Menopause," was funded by the National Health and Medical Research Council and the Victorian Health Promotion Foundation.
I take sole responsibility for the views expressed in this paper.

managing their lives at the menopause, and at the other end would be those who have no problems at all. Most women fall somewhere in the middle of the spectrum. The variation in the nature and the number of problems that these women can experience (both among different women and over time for an individual woman) leads to confusion, either when they try to explain to a doctor what the problem really is, or when they make repeated visits to a primary care physician with a different problem every time.

Given the range and diverse nature of women's experience of menopause, it is appropriate to refer to women's *problems* rather than to use the term *symptom,* although most doctors and many women refer to their problems as *symptoms.* A *symptom,* for example, a hot flash, is easily seen as being a single, isolated health problem that can be cured by prescribing the appropriate treatment. In midlife, though, problems are complex and seldom come singly, and treatment often presents problems.

Sociologists have a tendency to make things even more complicated. They rarely focus only on health problems but argue that these health problems can be understood properly only by taking into account whatever else is happening in women's everyday lives. There is a need to take women's physical health into account, but there is also a need to consider how well women are coping with their lives in general—whether they feel happy about where they are and what they are doing. Families are important as a source of difficulty, but they can also provide valuable support. A circle of supportive friends can make life a lot easier. Those of us with educational advantages, good jobs, or financial security undoubtedly have social advantages. Last, it is well established that society has a negative, stereotypical image of women in midlife (Greer 1991), and this undermines women's perception of themselves as socially valued beings. These factors all interact with the physical changes that come with the menopause. For this reason, it is preferable to talk about *problems* associated with *midlife,* of which menopause is a part.

To illustrate how the problems of women in midlife interact with and reinforce each other, two hypothetical cases are presented, one from each end of the menopausal spectrum. "Doris" is the Hamlet equivalent, with everything going wrong for her in menopause; "Mary" has the opposite experience and is able to see positive aspects of reaching the age of 50 years. These are two fictional cases with constructed characters in whom all the problems and pleasures are heightened for dramatic effect. In each case there is a general description of the kinds of problems they face, followed by comments on how HRT enters into the picture. Lastly, we look at women in the middle of the spectrum—those who are having problems but are battling their way through.

The Woman With Serious Problems

The danger for women who have serious difficulties in midlife is that they can see themselves as the source of their own problems. Alternatively, others can blame them for what is happening and suggest that they "pull themselves together." What is made clear in interviews with women in this group is that women may encounter problems as a result of sheer chance, including the family into which they are born, where they live, and the state of their physical health.

The effect of hormonal changes in midlife is also sheer chance. In the same way that some women have morning sickness when they are pregnant, some women suffer more from the hormonal shifts that occur during menopause. The ways in which women cope with these changes are, to some degree, a matter of personal choice. This choice, however, may be limited, sometimes even by personal choices women have made in the past and for which they may be partly responsible. Fortunately, women facing serious, disruptive problems in midlife were a minority in the La Trobe study (20 out of 150 women in a volunteer sample), but they are an important minority because they are most in need of help. Let us see how these problems play out in the case of the fictional heroine Doris.

Doris grew up in a poor rural family and left school at the age of 15. She married young and has spent her life as a wife and mother. In this role she has always unquestioningly put her family's needs above her own, especially because money has always been rather tight. When her husband lost his job at the age of 55, he could not find employment, and they are now very short of money. At the same time, her teenage son decided to give up his apprenticeship as a chef because he could not keep the hours that were required. He prefers to sleep late in the morning. For the past 6 months, the two men have sat at home in the family room all day, watching daytime television. Doris has had to provide them with snacks and meals. She is not at all sure that she likes having her space invaded in this way when she had become used to having the house to herself during the day.

The big advantage Doris has is a circle of supportive friends, and they suggested that she "get out of the house." Perhaps she could find herself a fulfilling job. She plays a pivotal role in various community and church activities, and they persuaded her that she had something to contribute beyond being a wife and mother. Like many midlife women, the problem Doris faced was that her feeling of self-worth was undermined as soon as she tried to obtain paid employment. When she applied for a position as a teacher's aide at a local school, they turned her down because, they said, she is too self-confident, and this would threaten the young teachers. She went home feeling that nobody cares about women when they are over 50—that they are placed on the scrap heap.

Doris is also having health problems. She has not had a period for 3 months, her feet are swollen, her ankles ache, and she has bad headaches. At times she has felt so depressed that she just wants to stay in bed and cry. On one occasion, she found herself driving her car and thinking that if she drove it into a tree, her problems would end. Alarmed at this experience, she went to her doctor and poured out a confused story of family and personal problems, hot flashes, headaches, and depression. Her doctor prescribed tranquilizers for stress and suggested that she get a job to take her mind off her family problems.

Unexpectedly, family relations improved. The male culture in the country town where she lives revolves around the achievements of the local (male) sports teams. Doris's husband and son are avid supporters of the local football team. Their team started the season badly but then, unexpectedly, started winning games and ended up at the top of the ladder. On the afternoon of the big game, Doris's husband went to watch it with his buddies at the local bar. Doris was happy to stay at home. As a distraction, she sat in the kitchen over a cup of coffee and tried to concentrate on Germaine Greer's *The Change,* but it did not seem to have any suggestions that made sense to her in her life. Her son was watching the game on television with a group of loud friends. Soon she became aware that the game was going against the local team. Each time a player dropped the ball, she felt hot all over. By the time her husband got home from the bar, she was feeling quite awful and very apprehensive. He was grimly furious, sat down at the kitchen table, and started going over their credit card accounts. When he found that she was missing three little yellow slips, he called her an "incompetent woman" and cut up her credit card. Doris had a hot flash that started at her feet, ricocheted off the top of her head, and bathed her body in heat. She felt her world closing in on her, reached behind her, and found a carving knife.

At this stage, Doris might, like Hamlet, "take arms against a sea of troubles" and do serious injury to some unspecified part of her husband's anatomy.

When charged with a malicious intent to harm, what should she plead in her defense? Perhaps her hot flash was the cause of the anger. Were she to blame her husband for abusing her over many years, she might quite justifiably become a cause célèbre for the feminist movement. Alternatively, she could blame the male sports culture or the state of the economy and the lack of employment opportunities for midlife women. Fortunately, unlike a trial judge, we do not have to apportion blame. We are free to accept that the most likely scenario is that all these factors acted together and proved to be too much for the restraint that she had exercised for the previous 35 years of married life.

Once we recognize the complex, interactive nature of Doris's problems, would we recommend that she take HRT? It is arguable that the prescription of HRT when she first went to the doctor might have prevented Doris's problems from becoming as bad as they did. It is worth noting here that, among the women interviewed, those with the worst problems were often denied HRT because, the women say, their problems were seen as "psychosomatic" or "neurotic." They were told to face up to the inevitability of aging or to pull themselves together. Here are two examples:

> . . . when I went to the local doctor when I first started getting all funny, the doctor just said, "Well, that is just part and parcel of life. Women have been going through this for centuries." (Carla)
>
> . . . You have to get past the doctor, who thinks you are neurotic when you ask for anything or tell them anything . . . . "Get out and get some more social life, take your mind off yourself, dear!" (Pauline)

In the La Trobe study, the women most in need of help were often given the least medical attention. But even if her doctor had prescribed HRT, would it have helped Doris? Even if it had cured only her hot flashes, that might have been enough to give her the strength to cope again with the many difficult problems that HRT could not cure—the personal, family, financial, and cultural problems. On the other hand, HRT might make matters worse. Doris might find that it did not cure her symptoms but complicated matters further by giving her sore breasts and making her headaches worse. She might gain weight, and she would have to have regular periods again. In her financial situation, she might not be able to pay for the pills or patches, let alone for the bone density scans and mammograms that are commonly recommended as part of the treatment. Doris may, like many women, feel as though she has lost the lottery and prefer to flush the tablets down the toilet.

The Woman With a Positive Experience

In a comedy about midlife, one would need a feisty heroine who negotiates whatever problems come her way successfully and with humor. Although there is a lack of characters in popular fiction who represent women with an extremely negative experience in midlife, there are fictional heroines who play this more positive role. Shirley Valentine, in the play and film of the same name (Russell 1988), is one, and she has acquired a considerable cult following among midlife women. She coped initially by conducting a dialogue addressed to the wall: "Wall," she says, "Who turned me into this? I don't want this. Do you remember her, wall? Remember Shirley Valentine?" When Shirley's husband goes too far, she joins a friend on a holiday to a Greek island and finds a (temporary) Greek lover who even kisses her stretch marks. Finally, her husband has to renegotiate their relationship, in Greece, on Shirley's terms. What Shirley managed was to make some space within which she could rediscover who she is and who she wants to be. Women like Shirley Valentine teach us about the positive aspects of what has been called the "midlife transition." My fictional heroine Mary has used her as a role model.

Compared with Doris, Mary has many advantages. She is well educated, has a good job, and is financially quite secure. When she reached the age of 53, she realized that she had not had a period for 3 months, so she went to the library and read up on the problems that were about to descend on her. However, nothing untoward happened. Her family is wonderfully supportive, and her husband believes that women in midlife should be given lots of TLC. He brings her tea in bed in the morning. When Mary hobbled downstairs one morning on stiff feet, her daughter saw it and made her sit down so that she could massage Mary's feet. Her daughter has now taken massage classes to be able to help her mother more effectively. This makes Mary's sore feet seem to be a minor worry in her busy day. With help and sympathy, Mary is, she says, gliding her way through midlife.

Mary has what women have looked forward to since Margaret Mead described her "postmenopausal zest." She has taken up Scottish dancing and goes off for weekends with her close circle of women friends. Together they make jokes about their physical changes. They have made a pledge to each other to cope with the hair growing on their chins: should anyone end up in the hospital in a coma, the others will sneak in with tweezers and pluck out the offending hair. They intend, they say, to be beautiful corpses!

Mary and her friends are aware of the sexual changes of midlife, but they know that the vaginal dryness associated with menopause may not be due to an estrogen deficiency but may well be caused by men's lack of sexual finesse. They tell jokes about it: "What is the midlife man's definition of a multiple orgasm? Oh, come, come, come!" Mary moved out of the marital bedroom when her son left home, and she has redecorated his room in a feminine style that entirely suits her taste. She invites her husband to join her there, and their sex life, she says, has improved considerably. On the other hand, she is relieved to find that she no longer feels dominated by the urges of her body. She says it will leave her free to spend her time developing her mind—and her stock portfolio. Her husband is, at any rate, very distracted with his business. On the other hand, she takes care of her appearance, but she does not tint her hair or try to emulate the latest Hollywood bimbo. In her view, she looks 20 years younger than most men her age.

Mary and her husband have the added pleasure in their lives of a beautiful baby granddaughter. Together they are exploring the joys of being able to indulge a baby without the responsibility of deciding how she is going to grow up. It is also a joy to them to see their daughter turn her talents to mothering as well as to her career as an engineer. Having a grandchild has made Mary more conscious of what it means to have children around who are loved and cared for. Recently she read Margaret Mead's description of her own experience of becoming a grandmother. The new baby, Margaret Mead said, made her see all other babies with a halo of light around them: "The known and loved particular child makes it possible for one to understand and care more about all children" (Mead 1989). This rang very true for Mary, and her response has been to become an active member of an international agency that looks after the needs of abandoned children. She feels as though she is earning a bit of a halo for herself as well.

Should women like Mary take HRT? This might seem like a ridiculous question, given that these women are gliding their way through midlife—or have taken action on a variety of fronts to restructure their lives in a more satisfactory manner. Again, things are more complicated than that. Some women are gliding their way through menopause because HRT has cured their symptoms, usually hot flashes. It is, of course, difficult to know what their lives would have been like without HRT. The problem for women gliding their way through midlife is, however, that they are often urged to take HRT not because there is anything wrong with them now, but because there might be in the future. They are urged to take HRT now to "store up credits" for themselves and their families in old age. One of the women interviewed expressed it very well:

> The chances are I'll live until I'm 90, and I don't want to be an old lady by the time I'm 90 who has bad bone density! . . . . I just want to be a healthy old lady. (Angela)

The problem is that a woman like Mary is going to have to wait a long time for these benefits, and there is uncertainty about whether they will eventually materialize. A woman whose mother is crippled, bent, and in pain may feel that anything is better than suffering in that way in old age, but Mary's own mother walks straight and tall at the age of 86. Mary herself is also not all that keen on menstruating until the age of 75 and running the risk of then discovering that it was, after all, not worthwhile. What Mary did was to read every article she could find on the problem in the newspapers. From these she learned that HRT could reduce the risk of heart disease and osteoporosis by 50%, and this sounded well worthwhile. She did, however, wonder what women would then die from instead.

Adequate information is a big issue in Mary's life. She belongs to that generation of women who took the pill when it first came out. She now knows that the doses of estrogen used in the first oral contraceptives were high in comparison with what is now acceptable. Because she took these early pills for 15 years, she is worried about the risk of breast cancer, but she also feels foolish for having taken her doctor's word that the pills were completely safe. As a result, she prefers to do her own research.

First Mary tried reading the medical literature on the subject, but it was very academic and seemed out of date, and she did not understand the terms used. In the media she then saw the report of a conference on the risks and benefits of HRT, and she decided that this report would be of immediate interest to her. The book, ordered through her local library, had an alarmingly vivid color illustration of a blocked artery on the cover. It told her that the results of studies on the benefits of HRT were "difficult to quantify" and it kept referring to what the results "suggest"; there was the problem of knowing whether HRT causes breast cancer (Samsioe 1991). It was clear that they were talking about averages, and she did not know how these averages would apply to her. This report did, however, tell her what she had not been able to establish from medical journals: she was amazed to discover that a 50% reduction in risk really means only that her life expectancy would be increased by 0.9 years and that some of this benefit would be lost if she did not take HRT over a long period of time. Her husband pointed out that this was the report of a conference and that the papers had therefore not been peer-reviewed for publication in a medical journal. This left her more than a little confused about where to turn for accurate information, but nevertheless she wondered why the media reports in the local newspapers did not take a similarly cautious approach to HRT.

Given these uncertainties, for Mary the benefits of HRT may not seem worth the risk. For other women, who can expect no immediate gain because they feel well, it may not seem worthwhile either. This is especially true if the HRT makes them feel ill. Anticipating a healthy old age may not seem to be a reasonable gain for suffering the side effects of HRT now. Most worrying is the problem of the "cascade effect"—when one intervention triggers a whole series of additional interventions to address the side effects of the first, which can finally harm the patient. Janet is one woman interviewed who narrowly avoided such an experience, despite the fact that her gynecologist was a personal friend.

> I just accepted [HRT] like a lamb. When I took it, I felt terrible. I'm not someone who suffers headaches, and I got this horrible pressure in my head . . . . I said, "Look, Rowena, I can't take it, I'm sure I can't take it!" She tried me on others, very, very low concentrations, different brands, and so forth. No good. Well, then [18 months later] she said, "I want you to have another bone density scan." And yes, my bone density had gone down a little bit, and

> she said "Well, I think at this stage I'm going to give you, I think you need a hysterectomy and then you'll be able to tolerate the hormone more easily." . . . And I thought, "I'm not prepared for this." So I went and got another opinion, and this doctor said to me, "I've never seen a woman less in need of a hysterectomy." I said, "Well, this is just exactly what I wanted to hear, thank you very much!" And off I went. But he also thought I should be on hormone replacement therapy . . . . Now, you see, I think I got caught up in that osteoporosis medical fad. And that is a very real thing, because they exert a great deal of pressure on you. (Janet)

The Woman Battling Her Way Through

Like Hamlet, Doris is an extreme case of a bad experience; like Shirley Valentine, Mary is doing well. Most ordinary women manage to get through their difficulties. Although it is not easy, they are successful because a few things go right for them or because they are more resilient in coping with the changes that take place. Evelyn Crouch, in Fannie Flagg's book *Fried Green Tomatoes at the Whistle Stop Cafe* (1987), is the fictional heroine who best represents this group. She has a considerable cult following.

Evelyn Couch has "gotten lost somewhere along the way" and has ended up fat and depressed about her gray life and her marriage to fat Ed. She is ready to kill herself. Then she befriends a wise and feisty 86-year-old woman who diagnoses Evelyn's problems as "a bad menopause" and works hard to help Evelyn regain a sense of self-worth. When at first Evelyn's efforts to be a new person fail, she gets angry. The action she takes is the stuff of delighted laughter from audiences of midlife women. In a memorable scene, she uses her car as a battering ram when two young women steal her parking spot. Aware that she cannot go on taking direct action, she turns to fantasy, inventing a new character for herself called Towanda, the Avenger. In this fantasy world she rights the wrongs of the oppressed, "machine-gunning the genitals of rapers and stomping abusive husbands to death, in her specially designed wife-beater boots" (p. 239). She even goes back in time to punch the apostle

Paul for telling women to remain silent. When Towanda invades Evelyn's real life, husband Ed sits up and takes notice:

> Later, as Evelyn was washing the dishes, Towanda was in the process of single-handedly blowing up the entire Middle East to prevent the Third World War. And so, when Ed yelled from the den for another beer, somehow, before Evelyn could stop her, Towanda yelled back, "SCREW YOU, ED!"
>
> He very quietly got up from his recliner and came into the kitchen.
>
> "Evelyn, are you all right?" (pp. 239–240)

The strategies that finally lead to Evelyn's reemergence as a highly successful cosmetic saleswoman are, however, multifaceted, including going to a "fat farm" and discovering the joy of religion. In the interview study, the strategies used by the women to address the problems that arise in midlife were similarly faceted.

Sometimes the problem is relatively simple but still distressing, like menstrual flooding. When medical help is ineffective, there is no option but to put up with the problem.

> Another time we stayed in a motel, and at 2 o'clock in the morning I woke up in this big pool of blood in the bed, although I'd had about five pads on to go to bed, and here I am, if you could have seen us, myself and my husband, washing this great big center of the sheet in the motel and then getting my hair drier out and drying this big circle, you know, in the middle of the sheet! And these are the things that you put up with. (Jenny)

Many women anticipate that midlife will bring them rewards for having been good wives and mothers in the past.

> You know, you manage to sort of hold this juggling act together with little kids, job, never having enough time, and just getting to the stage where there is a sense that you know and fall into place and you've got maybe the time to do what you wanted, your career, or to do things that you've always wanted to do, and never had time to do, and then suddenly your system starts fouling up again. So, that's the anger I think that a lot of women feel. (Bea)

They may be trapped not only by their own physical health but also by family circumstances, finding themselves at the beck and call of aging, dependent parents and the ongoing demands of adult children. As in the case of Mary, they can best take action to cope with these problems if they have access to reliable information about what is happening to them.

> . . . last Tuesday I thought I couldn't cope with anything more. Since then I have had another three to four good things happen to me and I am coping all right today. So I am just wondering how much of it is hormonal . . . . Last Wednesday I think I sat down and cried most of the day. Today I've got more worries but I am coping, so I don't know what it is.

In these circumstances, HRT may well prove to be of help. Evelyn Couch took HRT. It made her feel better and gave her an "enormous" orgasm. On the other hand, HRT on its own would not have worked; she also needed to address a number of other problems, which she could not have done without the help and strong support of 86-year-old Ninny Threadgoode. Among the women interviewed, there is also a strong emphasis on support from other women with whom experiences can be shared. These include talking about which of their problems are best seen as hormonal, which are best treated with HRT, and which are better addressed by more social means, like support from friends or community organizations. What these discussions offer women is support of the kind described by one of the women in the study:

> I mean, bit by bit we are working our way through these things, and we can say to one another, "Look, I really empathize with you, I truly understand how you are feeling, but just hold on, it will go, it will go!"

The Question of Hormone Replacement Therapy

Menopause is an experience that is surrounded by uncertainty. Women experience changes in their bodies and call themselves menopausal, but they are often not sure what is really going on. They see some of what happens as hormonal, and then HRT seems to be worth a try. HRT may help: it may remove hot flashes and, even if this is not the main problem in a woman's life, it may help her to cope with the other problems. On the other hand, HRT can make women feel worse. Either way, they may be concerned about the long-term risk of taking hormones. If women are experiencing no problems at all, if they are gliding through menopause, then the benefits of HRT depend on a real trust in the health gains in old age. These benefits are not so clear that women will generally continue with HRT if it has side effects that make them sick.

Should women take HRT or not? There is no clear agreement. HRT can help save the lives of some women who are coping with overwhelming difficulties, and it helps to make the lives of other women more bearable. It makes other women sicker than they were before. But women experience midlife in many different ways, and things are not always the same for any one woman. The answer may lie more in the woman's situation than in science, although science is also relevant. In general, the answer is as fuzzy as the symptoms of menopause: "Well, maybe, yes, but it all depends."

HRT is sometimes seen as the only way of confronting the problems of women in midlife. Let us return to the examples of Doris and Mary. If Doris had some of the advantages that Mary has, her health problems may stop and she may not end up feeling quite so desperate. Unfortunately, the focus on HRT as the "cure" for midlife ills has overshadowed any concern about the other problems of midlife, which HRT cannot address. Certainly HRT may help Doris cope with the changes in her life, but is this the best that we can do? Perhaps other interventions, like finding her a job or helping the family to see the effect they are having on her, may have a much more direct benefit. These interventions are preferable in a very important way: they are less likely to have long-term risks, including cancer. It is perhaps only when we see HRT as sometimes helpful and sometimes not that we will start dealing with other kinds of support, which would be much more helpful to women who are drowning in their problems in midlife, as well as those who are less afflicted.

References

Flagg F: Fried Green Tomatoes at the Whistle Stop Cafe. London, Vintage, 1987

Greer G: The Change: Women, Ageing and the Menopause. London, Hamish Hamilton, 1991

Mead M: Blackberry Winter: My Earlier Years. Gloucester, MA, Peter Smith, 1989

Russell WE: Shirley Valentine. London, Methuen, 1988

Samsioe G (ed): Cardiovascular Disease and HRT: New Perspectives. Papers presented at the 13th World Congress of Gynaecology and Obstetrics. Singapore, Parthenon, 1991

Chapter 2

The Controversial Menopause: An Overview

Lorraine Dennerstein

Menopause is a physiological event that occurs in all women. Menopause usually occurs in midlife, between 45 and 55 years, and most commonly at age 51 years. However, menopause may occur earlier or later. When menopause occurs before the age of 40 years, it is said to be early or premature.

There is no universal agreement on how to define menopause. The term *menopause* literally means "pause in menstruation." Its scientific definition is the last occurrence of menstruation, but this can be decided only after the fact. Also, because of frequent irregularities of bleeding at this time in a woman's life, it must be 12 months since a woman's last period to be sure menopause has occurred.

In a wider sense, *menopause* is used by laypersons, doctors, and researchers to refer to a much longer period of life, sometimes called the climacteric. This is a period of up to 10 years during which there is a complex transition that involves biological, psychological, sociological, and cultural factors.

The terms *premenopause, perimenopause,* and *postmenopause* are also used in various ways. In this book, *premenopause* refers to the phase in which women experience regular menstrual cycles and have not yet entered the menopausal transition; *perimenopause* is characterized by changes in menstrual frequency; and *postmenopause* refers to the phase that follows the final menstrual period.

That menopause is an important developmental phase influenced by specific sociocultural factors has been well documented. Thus menopause is both a social and a biological construct. Not surprisingly, viewpoints have become alarmingly polarized between those who perceive menopause to be a normal developmental phase occurring in the lives of all women and those to whom menopause is an endocrine deficiency disease.

From the clinical perspective, menopause may be accompanied by distressing symptoms, and it has increasingly been implicated in some major age-related diseases in women, particularly cardiovascular disease (MacLennan 1992) and osteoporosis (Wark 1996). Vigorous public and scientific debate accompanies many of these issues. Most women, aware of the controversy through the attention it receives from the media, seek a balanced discussion and explanation.

Normal Transition Versus Endocrine Disorder

In 1946 the World Health Organization defined health as a state of complete physical, mental, and social well-being and not merely the absence of disease or infirmity. Member nations agreed to a target of "Health for All by the Year 2000" and implicitly agreed to this positive idea of health. Yet a focus on symptoms, diseases, and disorders (indicators of ill health) continues to pervade much medical literature. This focus on pathology is equally evident in research on menopause, in which the overwhelming focus on pathology and medical treatments has led to increasingly vocal critiques of the apparent medicalization of a normal part of women's experience (Bell 1990; Greer 1991).

The contemporary Western medical description of menopause as "ovarian failure" or "estrogen deficiency disease" defines the midlife woman as sick and requiring treatment with hormone "replacement" therapy (HRT) to replace the declining production of estrogen by the ovaries. This view of menopause as a hormone deficiency disease began to appear in scholarly articles in the 1930s and was highlighted in 1966 by Dr. Robert Wilson's book *Feminine Forever.* He likened menopause to a deficiency disease similar to diabetes (Wilson 1966).

The alternative view, argued by, among others, Germaine Greer in her book *The Change,* is that menopause is a part of the life cycle, a normal developmental transition, a time for continued growth and development for meeting new challenges and developing new skills (Greer 1991). This transition may involve change or growth of self—biologically, psychologically, and socially. To define menopause in terms of health and illness gives it a medical meaning and changes its social meaning—as a marker of the end of the reproductive phase of a woman's life—to a medical meaning—hormone deficiency. Medical practice, in the form of HRT, is then necessarily used to correct the hormone deficiency, which is held responsible for problems occurring in mid- and later life.

Major disadvantages accrue from the medicalization of the menopause. For one, it reinforces the idea that women are controlled by biology in general and their reproductive systems in particular. The labeling of menopause as an illness may then preclude the woman herself, her friends, and her family from examining the other circumstances of her life that are contributing to her problems.

It is important to distinguish the differences between experiences directly related to menopause and those related to aging. The two are not necessarily synonymous. As a society, we are frightened of old age, and menopause is seen as a marker for old age in women. Our culture tends to have a negative picture of menopause and promotes the idea that women are a burden at this time of their lives. This attitude makes women more vulnerable to the view that menopause is a deficiency disease requiring HRT treatment.

The Changes

Biologically, the 10 years encompassing the menopause are those of a progressive change in ovarian function. After menopause, relatively low levels of the ovarian steroids—estrogen and progesterone—and high levels of gonadotropins are found, and the cyclical hormonal changes of the reproductive years are reduced. The extent to which other factors, especially social factors, interact to determine immediate and longer-term health outcomes has not been adequately assessed.

Psychologically, during menopause, a woman must deal with her changing internal hormonal environment, her loss of reproductive capacity, and the transition into mid- and later life. Socially, there are many problems confronting a woman in midlife, including adolescent rebellion and children leaving (or returning) home, confronting physical illness (of herself, her partner, or her parents), caring for sick members of the family, and marital stresses relating to midlife transitions.

Negative attitudes toward menopause have been shown to predict the later occurrence of symptoms (Avis and McKinlay 1991). Most women report feelings of relief or neutral feelings about the cessation of menses, and attitudes toward menopause become more positive as women pass through the transition (Avis and McKinlay 1991). Thus a positive change in attitudes toward the menopause and toward aging may have a beneficial effect on menopausal symptoms. Factors such as educational level, occupational status, income, and social network may influence the ways in which women adapt to the many changes occurring in the menopausal years.

Cultural factors, such as change in status accompanying menopause and stereotypical attitudes toward aging and reproductive roles, may also be influential. Menopause is as much a cultural experience as a physical one, and a woman's transition through this period of life is affected by society's beliefs, expectations, and customs regarding menopause and older women. Sandra Coney, in her 1993 book *The Menopause Industry,* points out that there are as many different types of menopause as there are cultures; although the cessation of menstruation is common to all women, symptoms can vary from culture to culture. Studies in Asia have shown that menopausal symptoms are not nearly as severe as those recorded in studies in the West (Avis et al. 1993). An early study among Rajput women in India showed that they had very few problems associated with menopause (Flint 1975). For these women, menopause was perceived as a reward. Whereas previously they had lived veiled and secluded in purdah, they could now leave the women's quarters and join in the men's talking and drinking activities. A later study of middle-class, educated women in Varanasi City, India, found many of these women to be bothered by hot flashes (Sharma and Saxena 1981).

Symptoms and Experiences of Menopause

Despite the ubiquity of menopause in Western societies, very little is known about the normal range of experience of this event and the factors that may affect it. Some women experience very few bodily or psychic changes, whereas others have their quality of life disturbed by symptoms that are claimed to affect many bodily systems. The most frequently experienced symptoms are hot flashes (or flushes) and night sweats. Some women find vaginal lubrication during sexual arousal more difficult with the menopause, which may affect sexual enjoyment. Irregular menstruation is common in the perimenopause, and problems with the urinary tract may become more frequent after the menopause. Osteoporosis, cardiovascular disease, and urogenital disorders have been implicated as long-term consequences of the cessation of ovarian endocrine activity associated with menopause.

Many middle-aged women seek information about what changes are usually associated with menopause. Before studies based on the general population were done, knowledge of menopause was based on a small proportion of self-selecting, predominantly ill women. Women who consult their doctors about menopause are not typical of women in the general population, and they can be expected to report more symptoms (Morse et al. 1994). Women who have had hysterectomies have also been found to have more severe symptoms overall than women who reach menopause naturally (McKinlay et al. 1987). Thus, studies of women seeking help at menopause clinics or from their own physicians often find a high level of symptoms. On the other hand, social scientists, who look at climacteric symptoms in a population at large usually find a lower level of symptoms. Studies of middle-aged women chosen randomly from the general population have been carried out in a number of European countries (Netherlands, Norway, Sweden), North America (United States and Canada), Australia, and Japan. Many of these studies have followed women over some years through the menopausal transition. The studies have used standardized, objective definitions of menopausal status, have used validated and reliable survey instruments, and have distributed questions relating to menopause in a list of other health-related symptoms. However, the studies have often excluded women who have had hysterectomies and sometimes those who are taking hormones for their symptoms, resulting in samples that are healthier than the general population.

The prevalence of hot flashes ranges from 0% in Mayan women to 80% in Dutch women (Oldenhave and Jaszmann 1991). Hot flashes and sweats are common in women throughout Europe and North America, and, although social factors in these countries may to some extent predict who is at risk, menopausal status per se seems to be the primary causal factor. Even so, a certain percentage of women report hot flashes many years before the menopause begins, and hot flashes reach their peak with the actual cessation of menses.

Ballinger (1985) found that both women seeking medical help for their climacteric symptoms and those around age 50 who were approached by researchers in a shopping center reported the same incidence of hot flashes (75%–80%) and vaginal dryness, but that those seeking help had more psychological and certain other symptoms, such as sweating, palpitations, and paresthesia. Oldenhave and Jaszmann (1991), of the State University of Leiden in the Netherlands, found that nearly 80% of Dutch women have experienced hot flashes; the highest prevalence was in those whose last menstrual period occurred between 6 and 12 months before the survey. These researchers found that hot flashes and sweating seemed to be related to the severity of nearly all other complaints. A survey of women recruited from an ovarian screening clinic at Kings College Hospital, London (Hunter 1992), found that 15%–25% of women had hot flashes before the menopause. As they reached the menopause, the incidence of hot flashes increased to 54%.

In Europe and the United States, the women most bothered by the climacteric are those in lower socioeconomic classes. In Asian studies, there are conflicting findings about the relationship of symptoms and social class (Punyahotra et al. 1997).

Most studies have focused on complaints rather than assessing the balance with positive aspects of health and well-being. The Melbourne (Australia) Women's Midlife Health Project included the use of a validated well-being questionnaire to measure positive aspects of psychological health. The first part of the Melbourne study was a cross-sectional survey of 2,000 Australian-born women who were residing in Melbourne and were between 45 and 55 years old. Women were interviewed by telephone, and telephone numbers were selected randomly from a computerized telephone directory database. A 70.6% response rate was achieved from women who were eligible and available for the study. Menopausal status was 17% premenopausal, 29% perimenopausal, and 19% naturally postmenopausal. An additional 22% had undergone hysterectomy with or without removal of the ovaries, and 21% of the sample were taking HRT.

The first objective of the study was to determine women's experiences of the natural menopausal transition. Although negative stereotypes of women in midlife abound, suggesting that middle-aged women tend to be depressed and irritable, this study, based on the general population, found that the majority of middle-aged women reported positive moods most of the time (Dennerstein 1994). Of the women responding, 55%–72% reported that most of the time they felt satisfied, clear-headed, useful, loving, optimistic, and good-natured—not exactly the stereotype painted of the miserable, distressed menopausal woman! Moods (positive and negative) were profoundly influenced by social factors (such as marital status, employment, education, attitudes to menopause and aging, and stress), lifestyle factors (such as exercise and smoking), and health status. All the women who were still menstruating were then invited into a longitudinal study in which women are followed annually for 9 years. Analysis of the first 4 years of data found that negative moods increased significantly in the 2 years after the final menstrual period (Dennerstein et al. 1997). Negative moods then began to spontaneously improve.

The number of bothersome symptoms reported in the prior 2 weeks varied significantly with the menopausal transition (Dennerstein et al. 1993). Premenopausal women were the least symptomatic, and perimenopausal women were the most symptomatic. Menopausal status was significantly related to hot flashes and sweats, which increased throughout the menopausal transition, and to general somatic symptoms, which were more frequent in the perimenopause. Although hot flashes are not troubling for the majority of menopausal women, a sizable group in this study (39%) reported hot flashes as bothersome. Some 13% of premenopausal women, 37% of perimenopausal women, and 62% of postmenopausal women reported having had at least one hot flash in the previous 2 weeks (Guthrie et al. 1996). Women who experienced more hot flashes were likely to have higher levels of follicle-stimulating hormone (FSH) and lower levels of estradiol (Guthrie et al. 1996) and to have a history of menstrual complaints. The reporting of bothersome symptoms was associated with factors similar to those affecting mood.

Studies of patients at menopause clinics in the United Kingdom, the United States, and Australia have reported a high prevalence of sexual difficulties and marital problems. Again, it is not clear how frequently these problems occur in the general population of middle-aged women and how any changes in sexual functioning relate to biological, psychological, and social changes occurring in midlife. Relatively few of the recent population studies of middle-aged women have inquired about sexual functioning. An early cross-sectional study by a Swedish investigator of 800 randomly selected women aged 38, 46, 50, and 54 years found that a decrease in sexual interest and in orgasmic and coital frequency correlated with menopausal status rather than with aging (Hallstrom 1977). Yet a U.K. study found no increase in the incidence of sexual problems associated with the occurrence of menopause per se (Osborn et al. 1988). Certainly there is a great deal of evidence that other factors, particularly relationship aspects and social variables such as social class, marital status, and educational level, affect sexual behavior. The biological changes of the menopause are associated with atrophic, or drying, changes in the lower urinary tract and vagina. These changes make some women more prone to problems such as infections, incontinence, and difficulty with vaginal arousal or lubrication, which can cause discomfort or pain with intercourse.

The Melbourne Women's Midlife Health Project (Dennerstein et al. 1994) found that over the previous 12 months most women reported no change in their sexual interest, 31% reported a decrease in sexual interest, and 7% reported an increase. Women least likely to report a decline in sexual interest were those who were premenopausal, had a high sense of well-being, were in paid employment, had 11–12 years of education, and had low levels of bothersome symptoms.

Two major long-term health problems have been linked to the occurrence of menopause. These are cardiovascular disease, which may result in heart attacks, and osteoporosis, or loss of bone density, which may result in fractures. Before menopause, women seem to be protected against cardiovascular problems to a greater extent than do men, but after menopause, there is a gradual increase in the incidence of these problems. Similarly, with menopause there is an increased thinning of bone. The role of menopausal estrogen reduction in the occurrence of cardiovascular problems and osteoporosis is currently the topic of much research. There is considerable debate about the role of administering estrogen to prevent these disorders later in life. The issues underlying the debate are detailed in the following chapters. In examining the possible role of HRT, it is important to keep the broad picture in mind—that is, endocrine change is one of many factors affecting cardiovascular and bone functioning. Other factors include genetic predisposition, smoking, alcohol, nutrition, and exercise. These factors are discussed in the following section and in more detail in Chapters 8 and 9.

Treatment Controversies

Women approaching and in midlife have been confronted in the past few years with a rush of information about menopause and the use of HRT. Yet HRT is not a new concept. Since the 1950s, women have been treated with various combinations of hormones after hysterectomy or for menopausal symptoms such as hot flashes and vaginal dryness. Recently, HRT has also been promoted as a preventive therapy for osteoporosis and heart disease.

Conflicting messages are creating uncertainty in some women, who have been made to feel they should be taking HRT but do not like the side effects, the pill taking, or the continuation of menstruation that sometimes accompanies HRT. The debate about HRT is currently focused on these risks and benefits. For some women, the positive effects of HRT are liberating. It can help control hot flashes and bladder problems. Estrogen creams can alleviate vaginal dryness and infection caused by fragile vaginal tissue (Coope 1996). However, many women using HRT complain of side effects, including fluid retention, nausea, weight gain, and sore breasts. Sometimes these effects are diminished when the dose of hormone is reduced or the type of hormone used is changed. Unusual bleeding patterns may be a problem and must be examined to be sure they are not caused by other complications. Overseas studies have found that among women using HRT, there is a higher hysterectomy rate and a greater number of gynecological procedures performed (Ettinger et al. 1988).

Women's experiences of HRT vary widely. Some will not consider it, others think it is wonderful, and some think it is good but dislike the side effects. A woman's decision of whether to use HRT is most often based on its immediate positive or negative effects rather than its possible future preventive effects.

Much of the promotional information about HRT ignores the potential risks associated with it, and information about the beneficial effects usually comes from research on women taking estrogen alone. Estrogen-only therapy is known to be associated with endometrial (or uterine) cancer (Weiss and Hill 1996); therefore, women are now more often prescribed estrogen in combination with a progestin. There is also evidence that estrogen is associated with an increased risk of breast cancer (Ewertz 1996) and gallbladder disease. There are not enough data on how the addition of progestins to estrogen therapy affects the risk of cardiovascular disease. Large clinical trials by the Women's Health Initiative are now under way in the United States, and it is hoped that they will answer some of these questions in the next few years.

Because not enough research has been done on these drugs, it is difficult to give women a clear picture of their risks and benefits. In the long term, patterns of disease are changing in our society. The incidence of heart disease is decreasing; that of breast cancer is increasing. This makes it even more difficult to assess whether HRT will have clear benefits in 15–20 years' time.

A case can be made for using HRT to treat hot flashes, night sweats, vaginal dryness, and some urinary problems. But even then, other factors are associated with reduced hot flashes and other symptoms. These include education, better health, fewer drugs, low stress, not smoking, exercising once a week, and having positive attitudes about aging and menopause.

We do not yet know whether HRT can prevent an increase in negative moods after menstruation ceases. However, other factors are known to be associated with better health and well-being, including living with a partner, absence of interpersonal stress, not smoking, exercising for health and fitness, and positive attitudes about the menopause and aging (Dennerstein 1996). Most of these factors are clearly within our control to do something about—for example, using techniques that lower stress (relaxation techniques, self-hypnosis, yoga, meditation). When the source of stress relates to ongoing marital or sexual problems, specific counseling may be needed to resolve these issues. Psychological aspects of the midlife transition and menopause are discussed further in Chapter 7.

The facts are simply not in yet, from prospective (or follow-up) studies or from large randomized trials, on whether taking HRT will decrease cardiovascular problems or reduce fractures enough to justify recommending this therapy to most women in midlife. The disadvantages or risks, such as an increased risk of breast cancer, still remain to be adequately documented.

This book attempts to sum up for women what is and is not known about menopause and HRT. HRT has a role for those troubled by disabling symptoms that are known to respond to it, and it may have a role for those specifically at risk for longer-term problems, such as cardiovascular disorders and osteoporosis. As part of the bigger picture, the other factors known to influence health are also discussed. Positive attitudes toward aging and menopause, healthy lifestyles—with no smoking, minimal alcohol, and adequate exercise and nutrition—and stress reduction can be used constructively by women to protect their health.

References

Avis NE, McKinlay SM: A longitudinal analysis of women's attitudes toward the menopause: results from the Massachusetts Women's Health Study. Maturitas 13:65–79, 1991

Avis N, Kaufert P, Lock M, et al: The evolution of menopausal symptoms. Bailliere's Clinical Endocrinology and Metabolism—International Practice and Research 7:17–32, 1993

Ballinger SE: Psychosocial stress and symptoms of menopause: a comparative study of menopause clinic patients and non-patients. Maturitas 7:315–327, 1985

Bell S: Sociological perspectives on the medicalization of menopause. Annals of the New York Academy of Sciences 592:1–488, 1990

Coney S: The Menopause Industry. Melbourne, Spinifex Press, 1993

Coope J: Hormonal and non-hormonal interventions for menopausal symptoms. Maturitas 23:157–166, 1996

Dennerstein L: In pursuit of happiness: well-being during the menopausal transition, in The Modern Management of the Menopause. Edited by Berg G, Hammar M. Lancaster, UK, Parthenon Publishing Group, 1994, pp 151–160

Dennerstein L: Well-being, symptoms and the menopausal transition. Maturitas 23:145–157, 1996
Dennerstein L, Smith AMA, Morse CA, et al: Menopausal symptomatology in Australian women. Medical Journal of Australia 159:232–236, 1993
Dennerstein L, Smith AMA, Morse CA, et al: Sexuality and the menopause. Journal of Psychosomatic Obstetrics and Gynaecology 15:59–66, 1994
Dennerstein L, Dudley E, Burger H: Well-being and the menopausal transition. Journal of Psychosomatic Obstetrics and Gynaecology 18:95–101, 1997
Ettinger B, Golditch IM, Friedman G: Gynecologic consequences of long-term unopposed estrogen replacement therapy. Maturitas 10:271–282, 1988
Ewertz M: Hormone therapy in the menopause and breast cancer risk: a review. Maturitas 23:239–246, 1996
Flint M: The menopause: reward or punishment? Psychosomatics 16:761–763, 1975
Greer G: The Change: Women, Aging, and the Menopause. London: Hamish Hamilton, 1991
Guthrie JR, Ebeling PR, Hopper JL, et al: Bone mineral density and hormone levels in menopausal Australian women. Gynecological Endocrinology 10:199–205, 1996
Hallstrom T: Sexuality in the climacteric. Clinical Obstetrics and Gynecology 4:227–239, 1977
Hunter M: The South-East England longitudinal study of the climacteric and postmenopause. Maturitas 14:117–126, 1992
MacLennan A: Hormone replacement therapy: the evidence on primary and secondary prevention of coronary disease—a gynaecologist's viewpoint, in Women and Coronary Disease. Edited by Kelly DT. Edgecliffe, Australia, Excerpta Medica, 1992, pp 23–31
McKinlay JB, McKinlay SM, Brambilla DJ: Health status and utilization behavior associated with menopause. American Journal of Epidemiology 125:110–121, 1987
Morse CA, Smith AMA, Dennerstein L, et al: The treatment-seeking woman at menopause. Maturitas 18:161–173, 1994
Oldenhave A, Jaszmann LJB: The climacteric: absence or presence of hot flashes and their relation to other complaints, in The Climacteric Hot Flush. Edited by Schonbaum E. Progress in Basic Clinical Pharmacology, Vol 6. Basel, Karger, 1991, pp 6–39
Osborn M, Hawton K, Gath D: Sexual dysfunction among middle aged women in the community. British Medical Journal 296:959–962, 1988

Punyahotra S, Dennerstein L, Lehert P: Menopausal experiences of Thai women, I: symptoms and their correlates. Maturitas 26:1–7, 1997
Sharma VK, Saxena MSL: Climacteric symptoms: a study in the Indian context. Maturitas 3:11–20, 1981
Wark JD: Osteoporotic fractures: background and prevention strategies. Maturitas 23:193–207, 1996
Weiss NS, Hill DA: Postmenopausal estrogens and progestogens and the incidence of gynecologic cancer. Maturitas 23:233–238, 1996
Wilson RA: Feminine Forever. London, WH Allen, 1966

Further Reading

Farrell E, Westmore A: The HRT Handbook. Melbourne, Anne O'Donovan, 1993
Greer G: The Change: Women, Aging, and the Menopause. London, Hamish Hamilton, 1991

CHAPTER 3

Hormones: What They Are and What They Do

Henry G. Burger

To understand the nature of hormones, it is necessary to think about how a complex system of organs and tissues such as the human body is controlled. We can think of our major body systems, such as the intestines, the kidneys, and the muscular system, as being controlled in two ways—one, the electrical signals from the brain, transmitted along nerves; and the other, chemical signals carried in the bloodstream. An analogy that may be helpful is to consider how a coach controls the activities of a football team on the field—the coach may use a telephone to relay messages, like the nervous system, or may send runners out to speak to the players, like the chemical signals of the hormone system.

Hormones, then, are chemical signals that originate in specialized tissues, the hormone-producing glands. These glands are different from the glands with which we are familiar—the ones in our necks and under our arms, which may become tender and enlarged if we have an infection. Those glands are not part of the hormone-producing system. The main glands that produce hormones include the pituitary at the base of the brain, the thyroid, the pancreas, the adrenal glands, and the ovaries and testes (see Figure 3–1).

Technically, the glands that produce hormones are called *endocrine,* a word derived from Greek roots meaning *to secrete internally.* Endocrinology is the science of hormones. In general, the body's chemical hormonal signals travel in the bloodstream and are transmitted only to the organs or tissues that are equipped with an appropriate receiver for the signal. One can use the analogy of a lock that only a particular key fits. The lock corresponds to the receiver in an organ or tissue; the key is the hormone, traveling around in the bloodstream and fitting only into locks in the so-called *target tissues.* Hormone control systems are often balanced systems in which the signal coming from one organ,

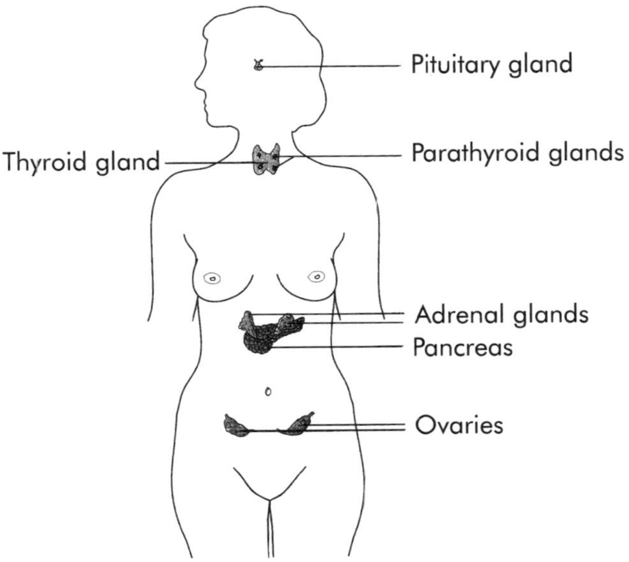

Figure 3–1. The hormone-producing, or endocrine, glands.

like the pituitary, is conveyed to another organ—for instance, the ovary—which may in turn produce a second set of hormone signals. Those signals will partly be transmitted to target tissues—for example, the breast, in the case of female sex hormones—but the signal is also received back at the pituitary gland so that if too much hormone is made by the ovary, it will damp down at the pituitary, and if too little is made, the pituitary will be activated. This system, called a *feedback system,* is characteristic of many parts of the hormonal system.

The Sources of Hormones and Their Effects

The Pituitary Gland

Hormones are made in specialized tissues, particularly the pituitary gland. This is an organ, about the size of a hazelnut, that is attached by a stalk to the base of the brain. The pituitary makes hormones that control the activities of a number of other members of the endocrine system. It in turn receives controlling signals from the brain itself. These signals are carried to the pituitary in a specialized system of blood vessels traveling between the base of the brain and the pituitary. Two hormones that play key roles in menopause are *follicle-stimulating hormone* (FSH) and *luteinizing hormone* (LH). These two hormones are involved mainly in controlling the functions of the ovary.

FSH could also be called *fertility-stimulating hormone* because it plays a part in the development of the egg and the structure surrounding it. If egg production is insufficient, the ovary fails to send the right signal back to the pituitary, and the amount of FSH in the bloodstream increases. This is what occurs after menopause, when no more eggs are left within the ovary and therefore the appropriate signal does not go back to the pituitary gland (Figure 3–2). Hence, when doctors measure the amount of FSH in the blood of women after menopause, they find concentrations 10 or 15 times higher than would be found during active reproductive life (Figure 3–2).

The second pituitary hormone involved in the control of the ovary is LH. This hormone could also have been called *ovulation-stimulating hormone* because it plays a role in the release of an egg in the middle of each monthly cycle. After menopause, LH reaches higher levels than those found during the reproductive years, but LH is not as useful a measure of the activity of the ovary as is FSH.

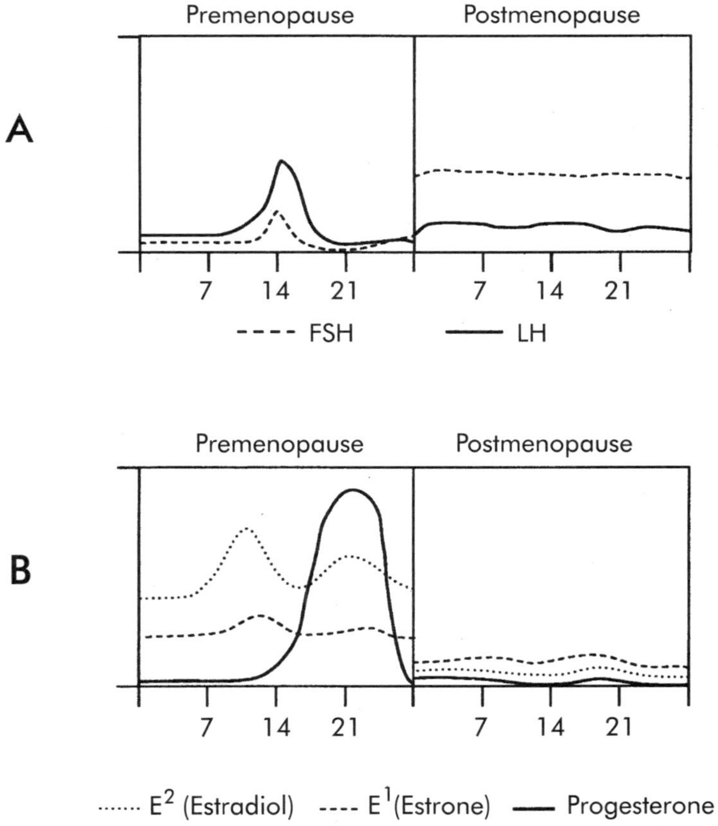

Figure 3–2. The main female reproductive hormones (A, follicle-stimulating hormone [FSH] and luteinizing hormone [LH]; B, estrogens and progesterone) during the normal menstrual cycle and after menopause. FSH levels are 10–15 times higher after menopause, estradiol is 90% lower, and progesterone levels are very low.

The Ovaries

Of the main hormone-producing glands, the ovary makes two general classes of hormones: the sex steroid hormones, of which the main examples are the estrogens and progesterone; and the peptide hormones, the main examples being inhibin and activin.

The best-known female sex hormone is estrogen, and the major active estrogen is called *estradiol.* Estradiol is normally produced by the structure that surrounds the developing egg. Its concentrations reach a peak halfway through the normal menstrual cycle, when they trigger the release of LH and hence ovulation (Figure 3–2). The levels of estrogen then fall abruptly but rise to a second and lower peak in the second half of the cycle.

Estrogen has many target tissues, but the one of particular relevance during the menstrual cycle is the *endometrium,* or lining of the uterus. Estrogen causes the endometrium to thicken and develop to prepare for the possible arrival of a fertilized egg. In recent years, it has been recognized that estrogens may elicit different responses from different tissues. Some estrogens derived from plants, as well as some synthetic (human-made) hormones, may have estrogen-like effects in some tissues (e.g., blood vessels and bone) and anti-estrogen effects in others (e.g., breast). These estrogens are called *selective estrogen receptor modulators* (see also Chapter 4). Some of these apparently paradoxical effects are due to the presence of more than one type of estrogen receptor, as well as to the existence of modifying factors that are specific to individual organs or tissues (Kauffman and Bryant 1995).

The second major hormone involved in the menstrual cycle is *progesterone,* also called the "pregnancy hormone." Progesterone is produced in the second half of the menstrual cycle, after an egg has been released (Figure 3–2). Progesterone also acts on the endometrium after estrogen has caused it to grow. Progesterone causes a marked change in the endometrium, making it ready for attachment of the egg and for its early nourishment. If no pregnancy ensues, the endometrium breaks down and is shed, with accompanying bleeding—the monthly menstrual flow.

In the past few years, we have also realized that the ovary produces another class of hormone, particularly *inhibin*. The main function of inhibin appears to be to act as a powerful feedback signal involved in the control of FSH (Burger 1993). It appears to be the combined lack of inhibin and estrogen after the menopause that leads to the very marked increase in the levels of FSH.

Therapeutic Uses of Hormones

When other hormone-producing glands of the endocrine system show evidence of decreasing production, it is customary for doctors to measure the levels of hormones in the blood to make a diagnosis. If the level of a hormone is low, then it is common to replace that hormone, either with the natural product itself, when that is available, or with a synthetic form of it. A good example of replacement with the natural hormone is the administration of thyroxine to patients with thyroid deficiency. In the case of the ovary, sex hormones are prescribed to treat symptoms linked to the withdrawal of estrogen in particular (Belchetz 1994). Hormones can also be used for long-term treatment if symptoms persist or to lessen the risks of heart disease and osteoporosis (see Chapters 2, 4, 8, and 10.) When hormones are used to treat disorders associated with the menopause, one can use either naturally occurring estrogens or synthetic estrogens for therapy. Progesterone itself is less available commercially than are the synthetic progesterones, called *progestins*.

The female sex hormones estrogen and progesterone are used in combination oral contraceptives. In this case, the estrogen is a synthetic estrogen, nearly always ethinyl estradiol. Although this is a much cheaper estrogen than the natural ones, it is not usually used at the time of menopause because, at least theoretically, it affects the liver more than the natural estrogens do and may more readily cause side effects as a result.

Examples of Hormone Action

To further understand how hormones work, a few examples can be given. One of the major products of the pituitary gland is growth hormone, which is essential for normal growth. In its absence, growth fails to occur; thus, a child with a deficiency of this hormone is much shorter than his or her peers. When growth hormone is administered, normal growth can be restored. A further example of hormone action is found in the case of a rather rare disease, acromegaly, in which too much growth hormone is produced. Acromegaly is characterized by overgrowth of organs and tissues.

An obvious example of the way estrogens work is found as a girl develops during puberty. At that time there is a height growth spurt that is closely linked with the beginning of increased estrogen levels in her blood. The breasts begin to develop, and fat is laid down in the characteristic areas found in the normal female. Pubic hair begins to appear, something that is certainly influenced by the female sex hormones, although it is also partly due to the action of male hormones. Estrogens thus "feminize" the female body at puberty, when they also cause growth in the size of the uterus and the vagina.

A further example of hormone action is increased hair growth on the body, a result of the secretion of male hormones (androgens). The male hormones are produced in all normal females by both the ovaries and the adrenal glands. If an excess of male hormone is produced, or if the hair follicles are unusually sensitive to the action of the male hormones, excessive hair growth can result.

Hormones and the Menopause

Estrogens

To put the matter of estrogen secretion and the menopause in perspective, we can think about the way estrogen is produced at different stages of life. In the first 3 months or so, surprisingly, estrogen is produced by a baby girl's ovaries, although its functions at that time are unclear (Burger et al. 1991). From about the age of 1 year onward, and until the beginning of puberty, the levels of estrogens in the bloodstream are too low to have significant effects. When puberty begins—and the signal for this is not well understood—the ovary gradually starts to produce greater amounts of estrogen. This triggers the production of growth hormone and leads to the beginning of the puberty growth spurt, usually at about the same time as the first signs of breast development occur. These two features of the beginning of puberty are both mediated by estrogen (Stanhope and Brook 1988).

During a woman's reproductive years, levels of estrogen fluctuate during each normal menstrual cycle, as described above. This fluctuation normally continues until the first indication of some irregularity in menstruation or in the amount of bleeding that occurs. The beginning of such irregularity—normally expected to occur about 4 years before menopause, is called the beginning of the menopause transition (McKinlay et al. 1992). The level of estrogen begins to fall at the beginning of the menopause transition and gradually continues to do so until 1 year or so after the last menstrual period (Figure 3–3). In fact, there is no clear break in hormone secretion at the time the last period occurs; therefore, hormone measurements just before and just after the last period are very similar (Metcalf et al. 1981). Estrogen levels continue to fall after the last period and reach very low levels by about 1 year later.

The results of this fall in estrogen levels may be quite variable. As indicated elsewhere in this book, many women experience few if any symptoms as a result of these falling estrogen levels. In other women, symptoms may be quite severe. They can be best understood if we consider the main target tissues for estrogen and how they react to the withdrawal of estrogen.

One important target tissue of estrogen is the brain itself. Much remains to be learned about the precise effects of estrogen on brain function, but one consequence of estrogen withdrawal is a change in the function of the part of the brain that normally maintains body temperature within very narrow limits. As a result of estrogen withdrawal, many women experience a *thermoregulatory disturbance*—an upset in the balance of the temperature-controlling system. This leads the body to believe that its temperature is too high and therefore to set in motion mechanisms for losing heat. This is what produces the hot flash, a disturbance lasting 3 or 4 minutes, which may occur many times a day or only very occasionally (Figure 3–3).

Many women also believe that during the menopause transition they suffer from problems with memory, self-confidence, and general well-being. It might be that these symptoms also reflect the withdrawal of estrogen from the brain, although this idea is much more speculative. Other important target tissues are those in the genital region, including the uterus, cervix, vagina, vulva, and base of the bladder and urinary passage. In some women, the result of estrogen withdrawal is a drying and shrinking of the vagina, which greatly decreases vaginal lubrication and makes intercourse uncomfortable. Disturbances of urinary function may also occur, particularly frequency of urination and recurrent infections of the urinary tract.

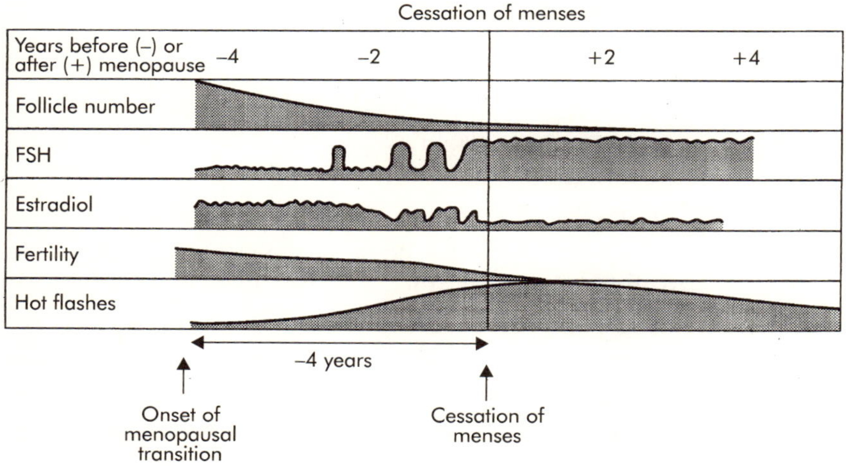

Figure 3–3. Some clinical, biological, and endocrinological features of the peri- and postmenopausal phases. The number of follicles produced by a woman's body gradually decreases as the final menstrual period approaches. Follicle-stimulating hormone (FSH) levels are raised intermittently before menopause and continuously afterward. Estradiol levels fluctuate before final menses and are low afterward. Fertility is already low as menopause approaches. Hot flashes commence before menopause and reach a peak in the first 2 years afterward.

Estrogen receptors are also present in the breast and the skin, and estrogen withdrawal may lead to some decrease in the amount of breast tissue and skin thickness. The normal female distribution of body fat is under estrogen influence, and a redistribution of body fat may occur after the menopause.

Estrogen withdrawal can have long-term effects on the bones and blood vessels, which also have estrogen receptors. Withdrawal of estrogen from the bones leads to an increased rate of bone turnover—the rate at which new bone is made cannot keep up with the rate at which old bone tissue breaks down. The resulting loss of bone tissue, if severe enough, can give rise to osteoporosis and the risk of fracture. Estrogen receptors are also present in blood vessels, and the withdrawal of estrogen may in turn be an important factor in the development of arterial blockage and heart attacks (Williams et al. 1990).

Progesterone

As the transition to menopause takes place and the menstrual cycle starts to become irregular, some monthly cycles are no longer characterized by the release of an egg—that is, they are cycles in which ovulation fails to occur. When that happens, progesterone is not produced, and the normal changes in the endometrium produced by progesterone do not occur. As a result, the endometrium may build up irregularly, leading to irregular bleeding. Thus, a consequence of progesterone withdrawal may be irregular and sometimes heavy bleeding. Progesterone protects the endometrium from excessive growth, and the increased frequency of endometrial cancer at this time of life reflects at least in part the loss of progesterone.

Androgens

A somewhat neglected aspect of the menopause has been the study of the changes that also occur in the levels of androgens at this time. All women produce androgens from both the ovary and the adrenal glands, which are located above the kidneys. The adrenal androgens decrease gradually with increasing age, a decrease not directly related to the menopause. The consequences of this decrease in adrenal androgens are somewhat unclear. The ovary produces small amounts of testosterone, as well as a related hormone, androstenedione. After menopause, the ovary continues to make quite significant amounts of both of these hormones. The total amount of testosterone in the bloodstream may not be affected much by the menopause, but the reduction in estradiol means that there will be less sex hormone–binding globulin in the blood, and therefore the testosterone will be more easily available to tissues. If the ovaries are removed, the amount produced is more than halved, representing the residual amounts produced by the adrenal gland (Hughes et al. 1991). There may be a case for replacing androgens in these women (Burger et al. 1987).

Summary

The menopause is a time of major changes in hormone levels. It is marked by reductions in the amount of the major female sex hormones estrogen and progesterone and a cessation of the production of the hormone inhibin. The pituitary gland responds by making much more FSH and some more LH. From a hormonal point of view, then, a typical postmenopausal woman has high levels of FSH, moderately high levels of LH, and very low levels of estradiol and progesterone, with some reasonable preservation of the normally low amounts of testosterone, which may be more available to target tissues than before menopause.

Hormone measurements are generally not useful in the assessment of a woman around the time of menopause, because, during the menopause transition in particular, these measurements may fluctuate very widely and thus do not provide reliable information (Burger 1994). Hormone measurements are occasionally of value after the menopause, particularly when diseases of the ovary or the adrenal glands are suspected.

References

Belchetz PE: Hormonal treatment of postmenopausal women. New England Journal of Medicine 330:1062–1071, 1994

Burger HG: Evidence for a negative feedback role of inhibin in follicle stimulating hormone regulation in women. Human Reproduction 8:129–132, 1993

Burger HG: Diagnostic role of follicle-stimulating hormone (FSH) measurements during the menopausal transition—an analysis of FSH, oestradiol and inhibin. European Journal of Endocrinology 130:38–42, 1994

Burger HG, Hailes J, Nelson J, et al: Effect of combined implants of oestradiol and testosterone on libido in postmenopausal women. British Medical Journal 294:936–937, 1987

Burger HG, Yamada Y, Bangah ML, et al: Serum gonadotropin, sex steroid and immunoreactive inhibin levels in the first two years of life. Journal of Clinical Endocrinology and Metabolism 72:682–686, 1991

Hughes CL Jr, Wall LL, Creasman WT: Reproductive hormone levels in gynecologic oncology patients undergoing surgical castration after spontaneous menopause. Gynecologic Oncology 40:42–45, 1991

Kauffman RF, Bryant HU: Selective estrogen receptor modulators. Drug News and Practice 8(9):531–539, 1995

McKinlay SM, Brambilla DJ, Posner JG: The normal menopause transition. Maturitas 14:103–115, 1992

Metcalf MG, Donald RA, Levesey JH: Pituitary-ovarian function in normal women during the menopausal transition. Clinical Endocrinology (Oxford) 14:245–255, 1981

Stanhope R, Brook CGD: An evaluation of hormonal changes at puberty in man. Journal of Endocrinology (London) 116:301–305, 1988

Williams JK, Adams MR, Klopfenstein HS: Estrogen modulates responses of atherosclerotic arteries. Circulation 81:1680–1687, 1990

Further Reading

Burger HG (ed): The Menopause. Bailliere's Clinical Endocrinology and Metabolism, Vol 7. Edited by Burger HG. London, Bailliere Tindall, 1993

CHAPTER 4

A Medical Perspective on Menopause

Diane Palmer

From a medical perspective, the question for women in midlife is not simply a debate about hormone replacement therapy (HRT). It is rather how best to assist women to maximize their health in midlife and beyond. Most women in industrialized countries such as the United States can expect to live about one-third of their lives after the menopause.

There are many questions that women ask about menopause, and, sensibly, they ask a lot more than whether they should take HRT. They want information about what is normal, what tests they should have, what they can do for themselves, and what treatment is necessary, appropriate, and available.

The Experience of Menopause

Menopause is a normal event, not an "estrogen deficiency disease." A woman's experience of menopause is influenced by many factors, all of which make each woman's experience of a normal physiological process unique—similar to the way in which every pregnancy is a unique experience. Events in a woman's medical and personal history, as well as the society and the culture she lives in, have to be considered in an overall assessment of her midlife health status (Kaufert 1996).

Menopause is a time when it is especially important for a woman to have access to information and answers to her questions. Only with such information can she make informed choices about her available options for her health care. It is appropriate for all women to look at and to choose some or all of these options to maximize their health. All women will benefit from the lifestyle modifications of stopping smoking, reducing alcohol intake, following good diets, and getting adequate exercise. These strategies need to be seen as complementary options to HRT, not just alternatives—it may be advisable to use them all.

The experiences of women during the menopause transition vary enormously and depend on many interacting factors, not just what is happening with their hormones (Dennerstein et al. 1993). The range of factors affecting a woman's menopausal experience include cultural and socioeconomic factors, employment, social support, stress, hormonal changes, and physical and emotional health. Some women have no symptoms at all, other than the cessation of their periods; others have very severe symptoms that greatly interfere with their lives. Some women who are having problems for other reasons may find even mild or moderate symptoms, added to other difficulties, too distressing to cope with. Research in several countries has found that women who seek medical help for symptoms are not necessarily those with the worst symptoms, but more often are those who are experiencing greater psychological stress than those who do not seek treatment (Ballinger 1988; McKinlay et al. 1992).

Hormone Replacement Therapy and Symptoms at Menopause

Women who have few or mild symptoms at menopause may need only to be reassured that what they are experiencing is common and normal. When symptoms are significantly interfering with daily life, it may be appropriate to look at specific treatments. Although the importance of good diet and adequate exercise must never be underrated, and although there are alternative forms of therapy that can provide some relief (see Chapters 8 and 9), HRT is the most effective and reliable form of treatment for distressing symptoms.

HRT as it is most commonly prescribed today is a combination of two hormones, estrogen and progesterone. It is the estrogen part of this combination that produces the beneficial effects. HRT in appropriate doses can provide relief from hot flashes and night sweats, usually within days to weeks. This is an enormous benefit for women who have really distressing symptoms. HRT provides relief from vaginal discomfort by increasing vaginal skin thickness and lubrication. The improvement in vaginal lubrication that HRT produces may in turn increase sexual pleasure and libido. The vaginal symptoms can take weeks to months to respond to treatment. The thickness of the bladder and urethral lining also increases after some weeks of estrogen therapy, and this often produces relief from symptoms such as a frequent or urgent need to empty the bladder or burning discomfort during urination. HRT may alleviate some of the symptoms associated with vaginal prolapse, but it will not cure the problem of prolapse.

HRT can also dramatically relieve the psychological symptoms of anxiety, depression, irritability, forgetfulness, and fatigue when they are directly related to the stress of symptoms and associated sleep disturbances. It may also have a significant effect when the relationship between physical and psychological symptoms is not so direct, but this effect is less predictable.

Some women taking HRT notice an improvement in dry hair, nails, and skin—this effect is due to the beneficial effects of estrogen on skin thickness. There is no proof, however, that HRT prevents wrinkles, and it is not an "elixir of youth" that prevents the normal aging processes. HRT frequently relieves the "crawling" sensation some women feel under their skin. It may also relieve the joint aches and pains experienced by some women during the menopausal transition, and it has been shown to have beneficial effects in some types of arthritis (although not in the most common type, osteoarthritis).

However, the symptoms at menopause are for the most part self-limiting—they usually get better with time. The average duration of hot flashes is 3–5 years, although occasionally they may last up to 10 years (rarely longer). Vaginal symptoms usually persist in the long term, although they are severe in only a minority of women.

When used for relief of symptoms, HRT may be needed for months or some years to help a woman through a difficult transition. For relief of vaginal and bladder symptoms, long-term HRT may be required (vaginal hormone cream can be very useful for this). When HRT is used for psychological symptoms, a trial period of 3–6 months is needed to assess its effect because of the likelihood that other contributing factors exist. When HRT is stopped, it should be slowly tapered off in case of a rebound of symptoms.

Hormone Replacement Therapy and Disease Prevention

In the long term, after menopause, the risks of osteoporosis and heart disease are increased. HRT can modify these risks to some extent.

Osteoporosis

At midlife and beyond, adequate calcium and exercise help to maintain the density of bones. Only HRT, taken from the time of menopause, has been repeatedly shown to stop the accelerated bone loss that occurs in most women after menopause. This benefit continues for as long as HRT is taken and thereby significantly reduces the risk of fractures. The incidence of hip fracture is up to 50% less in women who take HRT; the greatest benefit is observed in women who begin taking HRT close to menopause.

To prevent osteoporosis, HRT needs to be taken long term—possibly as long as 20 years. Once osteoporosis has been established, it is difficult to treat, and for this reason therapy to prevent the disease in those who are at risk is very important. HRT has also been shown, however, to have beneficial effects in established osteoporosis (Riggs and Melton 1992).

New drugs called *bisphosphonates* (e.g., alendronate, or Fosamax) have been extensively studied for their ability to prevent and treat established osteoporosis. These drugs have been shown to significantly reduce the rate of fractures and to increase bone density. These drugs are a suitable alternative for women with osteoporosis who cannot take HRT (Liberman et al. 1995).

Heart Disease

As women age, they face an increased risk of death from heart disease (coronary artery disease). This is thought to be due in part to the lack of the protective effect of estrogen after menopause. Estrogen has been shown to have beneficial effects on blood fats—increasing the levels of "good" cholesterol (high-density lipoprotein, or HDL) and decreasing the levels of "bad" cholesterol (low-density lipoprotein, or LDL). Estrogen also reduces the formation of blood vessel atherosclerosis (plaques causing narrowing of the blood vessels) and increases blood flow. It has been shown that women who take estrogen as HRT have a reduced rate of death from heart disease. This effect is even more marked in women who are at high risk of arterial disease (Lobo and Speroff 1994).

The Value of Hormone Replacement Therapy

HRT is very effective therapy for the relief of distressing symptoms around the time of menopause, but it should be part of an overall approach to maximizing health. This approach should also include diet, exercise, and other appropriate lifestyle changes.

In the longer term, HRT reduces the risk of osteoporotic fracture, most significantly in those at increased risk. There are many questions about the best ways of defining who these women are. We can identify some but not all of them on the basis of family history, personal history, and examination (see also Chapter 8), but the only reliable way is an assessment of bone density (measuring bone thickness by a form of X ray).

Bone density tests, for medical and economic reasons, have to be used in a selective way. Most doctors suggest the use of these tests if a woman has significant risk factors for osteoporosis or if it is going to make a difference in a woman's medical treatment—for example, if a decision to use HRT would be based on the result. HRT should be considered long-term therapy for women who are at significant risk of osteoporosis or for those with established osteoporosis.

Defining who is at significant risk of heart disease is similarly difficult. Many physicians now recommend HRT after a heart attack as preventive therapy against another attack. Women who are known to be at increased risk of heart disease for another reason—for example, those who have had premature menopause (before age 40)—are well advised to take HRT on the basis of reduction of heart disease risk alone.

The use of HRT is controversial for women who are not symptomatic and who are not known to be at increased risk of heart disease or osteoporosis. Some medical authorities believe that the potential benefits of preventing heart disease and osteoporosis outweigh any risks and recommend it for all women. Others are more conservative and recommend it only for women having symptoms of menopause or for those known to be at increased risk of future problems.

The selective estrogen receptor modulators (SERM) are a new development that is currently the subject of extensive clinical research. These are a series of compounds with estrogen-like and anti-estrogen properties. They are estrogen-like in that they attach to estrogen receptors in the cardiovascular system and bone, but they are estrogen antagonists in the way they behave with estrogen receptors in the breast and uterus. These substances (e.g., raloxifene), which are shortly to be released, hold promise for a protective effect against cardiovascular disease and osteoporosis, particularly for women at risk of, or fearful of, breast or uterine cancer (Kauffman and Bryant 1995).

Methods of Using Hormone Replacement Therapy

HRT is most commonly given as two hormones, estrogen and progesterone. Estrogen is given as a daily tablet or a twice-weekly patch that is stuck on the buttock or upper thigh, or as a 3- to 6-month implant that is inserted under the skin through a small incision. This estrogen replacement is designed to provide blood levels of estrogen like those of the first 2 weeks of a normal menstrual cycle. This level provides relief from symptoms and protection for bones and blood vessels.

The way estrogen is used for HRT is quite different from its use in oral contraceptives. The pill contains greater doses of stronger types of estrogen to prevent the ovary from releasing eggs. The estrogen used in HRT is sometimes described as "natural estrogen" because it more closely resembles the estrogen produced by the human ovary and is metabolized more easily by the liver than are the estrogens used in oral contraceptives. Tables 4–1 and 4–2 list the different types of HRT and average doses.

Progesterone (or its synthetic form, progestin) is given in addition to estrogen. When given with estrogen, progesterone counteracts the effect of estrogen on the endometrium (the lining of the uterus) by preventing its overgrowth. Progesterone is not needed in women who have had a hysterectomy, but it does still need to be prescribed for those who have had an endometrial ablation (removal of the lining of the uterus). It is most often given in tablets for 12 days a month, after which a withdrawal bleed (period) occurs in most women. This type of HRT is called *cyclical therapy.* About 10% of women who take this type of therapy do not have periods—this means that the lining of the uterus is thin and is of no concern. Progesterone can also be given daily as *continuous combined therapy.* In most women, this therapy does not produce periods after about a year, because the endometrium becomes quite thin. However, this type of therapy can cause troublesome, erratic bleeding in the first few months of therapy, especially if a woman is not long past menopause.

HRT may sometimes be started before menopause (while a woman is still having periods) if she starts to have distressing symptoms before her last period occurs. HRT can also be started some time—even many years—after menopause for symptom relief or to maintain bone density, although it has its most beneficial effect

Table 4–1. Average symptom-relieving dosages of estrogens

Estrogen	Average symptom-relieving dosage
Oral	
Estradiol valerate	2 mg/day
Piperazine estrone sulfate	1.25 mg/day
Conjugated equine estrogens	0.625 mg/day
Micronized estradiol	2 mg/day
Transdermal	
Estradiol patch	50 μg (for 3 days)
Subcutaneous	
Estradiol	50 mg/6 months
Vaginal	
Estradiol tablets	25 μg 2 times/week
Conjugated estrogen cream	2–4 g 2 times/week
Estriol cream	0.5 g 2 times/week

Table 4–2. Dosages of progestins for endometrial protection

Progestin	Regimen	
	12–14 days	Continuous
Medroxyprogesterone acetate	5–10 mg	2.5–5 mg
Norethisterone	0.7–1.25 mg	N/A
Norethisterone acetate	N/A	1 mg
Levonorgestrol	0.06 mg	0.03–0.06 mg
Cyproterone acetate	2 mg	1 mg

on bone when started close to menopause.

The type of HRT that has been studied and researched the most is oral HRT, as estrogen alone or combined with progestin (cyclical therapy). The non-oral forms of estrogen (the patch or implant) have been demonstrated to be as effective as the oral form in relieving symptoms. Short-term studies on the estrogen patch have shown it to have beneficial effects on bone density, which probably means that the risk of fracture is reduced in the long term (Garnett et al. 1991). Non-oral estrogen has a less marked beneficial effect on blood fats, but the other beneficial effects of estrogen on blood vessels and blood flow are not thought to be related to the way estrogen is taken. It is anticipated that the long-term effects of the estrogen patch against heart disease are likely to be the same as those of tablets (Cheang et al. 1994). Similarly, continuous combined therapy has been demonstrated to be effective as symptom relief. Studies on its long-term benefits are in progress, and so far the results confirm its beneficial effects on bone density and blood fats.

Occasionally, androgen therapy is given in addition to estrogen and progesterone therapy. Androgens are given in the form of testosterone, which can be administered as an implant or as an injection. Testosterone therapy may produce an improvement in libido that has remained unchanged by estrogen therapy, especially in younger women who have reached menopause prematurely or who have had both ovaries removed. Testosterone also has beneficial effects on bone density (Burger et al. 1987).

While taking HRT, a woman requires no specific examinations. Like all women, she should conduct regular breast self-exams and have a Pap smear every 2 years. Mammograms are now recommended every 2 years for all women over age 50 in order to reduce the risk of death from breast cancer. Because of their fluctuating nature, hormone tests are very rarely of value in assessing the need for, or the effect of, HRT (see Chapter 3).

Side Effects of Hormone Replacement Therapy

The most common side effect of HRT is the recommencement of periods, or withdrawal bleeding. Although the first bleed after beginning HRT may be heavy, periods while taking HRT are, for most women, increasingly light. When this is not the case, heavy periods usually become lighter with a change in medication. Other side effects occur in only a minority of women and, again, usually improve with medication changes.

It can take up to 6 months to find the right medication for an individual woman. Nausea can occur in the first month or two of therapy but usually goes away by itself or, if not, improves with a non-oral (patch or implant) form of estrogen. Breast tenderness is also usually transient and is less bothersome if the HRT dose is increased slowly. There is no significant average weight gain in populations of women who take HRT—some studies have shown that HRT users are in fact thinner than nonusers—but occasionally there are women who gain significant weight while taking HRT. Symptoms like those of premenstrual tension can be a problem in 10%–15% of women. They are usually related to the progesterone phase of therapy and can usually be helped with changes in therapy. Although side effects are not serious health problems, in some women they can be intolerable, and these women may be unable to take HRT.

Risks of Hormone Replacement Therapy

When hormone therapy was first used some 30 years ago, estrogen was given without progesterone. The increased incidence of cancer of the endometrium, which is due to the continuous stimulating effect of estrogen, is prevented by the addition of progesterone.

There is some argument about whether the addition of progesterone counteracts some of the beneficial effects of estrogen. It appears that there is no adverse effect on bone density maintenance, and some progestins have an additional beneficial effect. But some progestins theoretically have an opposing detrimental effect on blood fats. The recent U.S. Postmenopausal Estrogen/Progestin Interventions (PEPI) Trial found that estrogens given alone had the most optimal effect on blood fats. The most favorable regimen tested for women who still have a uterus was conjugated equine estrogen with cyclic micronized progestin (PEPI Writing Group 1995). Also, the beneficial effect of estrogen on cardiovascular disease is thought to occur in ways other than its effect on fat metabolism; therefore, it is anticipated that long-term effects of combined therapy on heart disease will be as beneficial as those of estrogen alone. A recent U.S. follow-up study of women enrolled in the Nurses Health Study found that those who took progestin as well as estrogen had a marked decrease in the risk of major coronary disease compared with women who did not use HRT. There was no effect on the risk of stroke (Grodstein et al. 1996).

The question of breast cancer and its relation to HRT is frequently mentioned, and it is difficult to answer simply. The results of research are somewhat conflicting, but they should become clearer with increasing experience. It is clear, however, that any increase in risk is quite small—if, in fact, the increase in risk is real and not merely due to the fact that women taking HRT are more closely screened for breast cancer. The risk conferred by taking HRT is less than the risk conferred by having a close relative with breast cancer, which doubles risk from 1 in 14 to 1 in 7. It is thought that HRT may alter the risk from 1 in 14 to perhaps 1 in 10, although it is still unclear whether this estimate is affected by length of use, type of HRT, and the presence of other risk factors for breast cancer. It has also been demonstrated that women who get breast cancer while taking HRT are likely to survive longer than those who have not taken HRT—perhaps related to earlier discovery and treatment of the disease. Most authorities believe that there is little or no risk associated with the use of HRT in the short term—up to about 8 years. After this period, there may be a small increase in risk (Colditz et al. 1993). A large cohort study in the United States involving over 422,000 women found no increased risk of fatal breast cancer among those who used estrogen therapy; in fact, there was a reduced risk for those who had ever used estrogen (Willis et al. 1996).

Other risks associated with HRT include potential worsening of liver disease and activation of systemic lupus erythematosus. Both of these risks are based on similar effects reported with the oral contraceptive pill. Women who have a personal or family history of blood clots may need special tests before commencing HRT to ensure that they will not have a recurrence of clots from taking HRT. Occasionally, gallstone disease may be worsened by HRT.

Summary

HRT is effective therapy for symptomatic women at the time of menopause. For women at increased risk of osteoporosis and cardiovascular disease, long-term HRT reduces those risks. Its use in women without symptoms and at low risk of long-term problems is controversial, but some of those women choose to use HRT. The decision to use HRT should finally be that of the individual woman after she has access to the information she needs to make her own choice.

References

Ballinger SE: Psychosocial stress and symptoms of menopause: a comparative study of menopause clinic patients. Maturitas 7:315–327, 1988

Burger H, Hailes J, Nelson J: Effect of combined implants of oestradiol and testosterone on libido in post menopausal women. British Medical Journal 302:936–937, 1987

Cheang A, Sitruk-Ware R, Samsioe G: Transdermal oestradiol and cardiovascular risk factors. British Journal of Obstetrics and Gynaecology 101:571–581, 1994

Colditz GA, Egan KM, Stampfer MJ: Hormone replacement therapy and the risk of breast cancer: results from epidemiologic studies. American Journal of Obstetrics and Gynecology 168:1473–1480, 1993

Dennerstein L, Smith AMA, Morse C, et al: Menopausal symptoms in Australian women. Medical Journal of Australia 159:232–236, 1993

Garnett TJ, Savval M, Studd JW: Osteoporosis prevention with oestrogen and progestogen, in Menopause and Hormonal Replacement Therapy: Facts and Controversies. Edited by Sitruk-Ware R. New York, Marcel Dekker, 1991, pp 247–256

Grodstein F, Stampfer MJ, Manson JAE, et al: Postmenopausal estrogen and progestin use and the risk of cardiovascular disease. New England Journal of Medicine 335:453–461, 1996

Kaufert PA: The social and cultural context of menopause. Maturitas 23:169–180, 1996

Kauffman RF, Bryant HU: Selective estrogen receptor modulators. Drug News and Practice 8(9):531–539, 1995

Liberman UA, Weiss SR, Karpf DB: Effect of oral alendronate on bone mineral density and the incidence of fractures in postmenopausal osteoporosis. New England Journal of Medicine 323:1437–1443, 1995

Lobo RA, Speroff L: International consensus conference in postmenopausal hormone therapy and the cardiovascular system. Fertility and Sterility 61:592–595, 1994

McKinlay S, Brambilla DJ, Posner JG: The normal menopause transition. Maturitas 14:103–115, 1992

Postmenopausal Estrogen/Progestin Interventions Trial Writing Group: Effects of estrogen or estrogen/progestin regimens on heart disease risk factors in postmenopausal women. Journal of the American Medical Association 273:203–208, 1995

Riggs BL, Melton LJ: The prevention and treatment of osteoporosis. New England Journal of Medicine 327:620–627, 1992

Willis DB, Calle EE, Miracle-McMahill HL, Heath CW: Estrogen replacement therapy and risk of fatal breast cancer in a prospective cohort of postmenopausal women in the United States. Cancer Causes and Control 7:449–457, 1996

CHAPTER 5

Why Hormone Replacement Therapy Is a Social Issue

Julia Shelley

Clearly, hormone replacement therapy (HRT) has become a social issue rather than a purely medical one. The appearance of articles in daily newspapers and the range of discussion in a variety of magazines suggest that there is a story in HRT. They also indicate that there is at least some level of controversy about its use that is generating discussion and debate in the general community. Why is this true? There are a range of influences that together form the basis of the debate about HRT. In this chapter a number of these influences are identified:

- Features of the generation of women now approaching the menopausal transition,
- The manner in which segments of the medical profession view menopause, and

- New research findings on the long-term effects of HRT and how they are interpreted by the scientific and medical community and the women's health community.

In this chapter, I examine the concept of a social agenda underlying much of the medical and scientific agenda regarding HRT. By looking at the social agenda in light of some of the scientific findings on HRT, we can develop a clearer picture of why HRT is a social issue.

Why the Interest in HRT?

It is worth noting that hormones of various kinds, including those marketed today as HRT, have been prescribed for hot flashes, and for other symptoms thought to be related to the menopause, since the 1940s. So, clearly, one of the questions we need to ask is, What has changed to make HRT an issue now, when it has been in use for so long?

Several things have changed. Women's lives have changed, what is known about HRT has changed, the way our society views scientific research has changed, and the way women patients interact with the medical profession has changed. Let's look at each of these in turn.

There can be little doubt that women are enormously interested in HRT and that this interest is one of the driving forces behind the HRT issue. The generation of women now reaching menopause is in many ways the product of the ways society generally has changed in recent years. These women are used to exercising some control over their domestic, social, and working lives. Women work—out of necessity and out of interest. Many are still working during their menopausal years. Women in this generation are less likely to suffer in silence—to accept that "it's all in your head, dear" or that "it's the change of life—so you just have to grin and bear it." Many women are saying "I don't want my life disrupted by menopause, and I will make sure that it is not"—so they ask for, and take, HRT.

Women in this generation have witnessed both the good and the harm that modern medical practice can do. Often, women are aware that they have a choice about their health care and their medical treatment. Increasingly, women ask questions about the possibilities available to them and seek information about how a particular problem or event can be approached. They are now seeking information about menopause and other aspects of health in mid- to later life, and hence about HRT.

It is also a generation that has listened to and acted on the messages that indicate that persons' lifestyles and behavior can affect their health, in both the short and the long term. Changes in diet, increasing exercise, controlling weight, and stopping smoking as ways of reducing the risk of heart attack and some cancers are familiar to many of us. Preventive health messages such as "take control of your own health" and "prevention is better than cure" have made their impact. Many women are open to suggestions about how to have a healthier older age, and there is a considerable amount of evidence suggesting that HRT may be one way of achieving a longer and healthier life.

Although many women consider menopause a natural transition, with which they cope in the same way they cope with many other fluctuations in their lives, in recent years doctors have increasingly come to consider menopause as a health problem, even as a disease. Menopause is viewed as a condition marked by the "failure" of the ovaries, leaving women in an "estrogen-deficient" state. By considering menopause in this way, they suggest that it is undesirable and indeed dangerous for women, rather than a normal phase of the life cycle. Hence, it is desirable that women be treated—and the treatment of choice is HRT.

The New Potential of HRT

As mentioned earlier, HRT has been prescribed for hot flashes for many years. When used for this purpose, it is often taken for relatively short periods of time, maybe a year or two, to ease women's path through the menopausal transition. Research findings released in the past few years have suggested that there are major benefits to be gained from HRT that go far beyond the control of hot flashes.

Much of the medical and scientific literature is now suggesting that HRT can prevent osteoporosis and heart disease if it is taken for long periods of time—for at least 10–15 years following menopause, but possibly for the rest of a woman's life (see Wark 1996 and Barrett-Connor 1996 for detailed literature reviews in these areas). These findings have led to HRT being heralded as a major breakthrough in the prevention of some very common and very serious conditions of older age—illnesses that are responsible for many deaths and much misery for older women.

It is not a great surprise, then, that HRT is being so heavily promoted—its known benefits plus its newfound potential benefits look very attractive. Why, then, should we not embrace it wholeheartedly? There are several reasons—questions about HRT that are explored in the next section: How good is the scientific evidence on HRT? Are health benefits the only (or even the main) agenda behind the promotion of HRT? How sure are we that the benefits of HRT will be delivered?

The concerns expressed in the following sections are about the possible effects of long-term use of HRT for preventive purposes. When used over relatively short periods (less than 5 years) to ease the effects of hot flashes and other menopausal symptoms, HRT has been shown to be quite effective; the benefits are clear and the risks fairly low.

The Scientific Basis for the Long-Term Use of Hormone Replacement Therapy

In this section, I consider the research that has led to all the interest in HRT for prevention of osteoporosis and heart disease and that has also indicated some of the risks and side effects of the therapy. Three aspects are examined:

1. What the research does not tell us about HRT,
2. How the studies that have been done are likely to have overestimated the benefits and underestimated the risks, and

3. The way in which the risks and benefits are put together pays little attention to women's views.

Current consensus suggests that HRT can reduce the risk of heart disease by almost half (Stampfer and Colditz 1991) and reduce the risk of hip fractures caused by osteoporosis by about a quarter (Grady et al. 1992). On the other hand, it is thought that HRT also increases the risk of breast cancer, but only slightly and after some years of use (about a 30% increase after 8–10 years) (Steinberg et al. 1991). When these findings are put together, they indicate that long-term treatment with HRT increases a 50-year-old woman's life expectancy by about 11 months (Grady et al. 1992). For women who already have a history of heart disease, the increase in life expectancy may be about 2 years.

What We Do Not Know About Hormone Replacement Therapy

The first aspect of the research findings is that they are almost all based on U.S. studies of women taking estrogen—in many cases, after a hysterectomy. Women who have not had a hysterectomy are usually prescribed combined hormone therapy—that is, the two hormones estrogen and synthetic progesterone, or progestin. There have been no long-term studies showing the effects of combined hormone therapy on heart disease. However, on the basis of what we know about progestins, it is thought that this type of hormone might slightly reduce the benefits of HRT to the heart (Grady et al. 1992). Second, there have been no long-term studies looking at whether the benefits of HRT are the same if estrogen patches rather than tablets are used.

Why the Research May Exaggerate the Benefit and Underplay the Risks

In many countries, there are strict laws and regulations about the testing, marketing, and promotion of pharmaceutical drugs to ensure that they are safe and are used for the purposes for which they are intended. A requirement for most new drugs is that their safety and efficacy must be tested by a scientific study known as a *randomized controlled trial*. This is the "gold standard" of drug testing. It allows the effects of a drug to be tested under closely controlled conditions rather than just by observation. This ensures that most other possible explanations for any observed effect have already been ruled out and the true effect of the drug can be measured.

Because both estrogen and progestins have been in use in various forms for so many years, their effect on osteoporosis and heart disease have never been studied in randomized controlled trials. Rather, their effects have become apparent from observing what happens to women who have taken estrogen for many years and for a variety of reasons. It is possible—indeed, likely—that just observing the impact of HRT in this way will have produced different results than those that might have been observed in a randomized controlled trial.

As I have already mentioned, most of the research on HRT has been carried out in the United States. In North America, it has been well documented that women who take HRT are much healthier than those who do not—they are of higher social class and have better health care and health practices associated with a low risk of heart disease, like good diets and lots of exercise. They have Pap tests and mammograms and other health checks—in other words, they are different from women who do not take HRT (Barrett-Connor 1991). What this means is that it is quite possible that these women would have had lower rates of heart disease even without the HRT.

It is important, also, to consider who has been included in the research and who has not. For a number of reasons, women who have a high risk of heart disease or breast cancer are likely not to have been included in research on HRT. Previous research experience with the oral contraceptive pill meant that women with a high risk of heart disease were often not prescribed HRT because it was assumed that it would increase the risk of stroke in the same way the pill does, especially among smokers. Similarly, fears about breast cancer and the pill meant that many women with a family history of breast cancer were not prescribed HRT (Barrett-Connor 1994).

Although most women who are prescribed HRT take it for only a very short time (less than 1 year), the research findings on the long-term effects of HRT are based on the experience of those relatively few women who have taken hormone therapy over several years. It has been shown in a number of research studies that those who take a recommended medication have lower rates of heart disease than those who do not follow the recommendation, even when the medication is a "sugar" pill or placebo used in a randomized trial. Whether the lower rate of heart disease among women taking HRT is the same phenomenon, due to some unknown characteristic of the women who have used HRT for long periods of time, rather than the HRT itself, is a possibility that researchers are as yet unable to discount (Petitti 1994). Together, this means that it is likely that the research findings have overstated the benefits on heart disease and underestimated the effect on breast cancer.

U.S. researchers and health authorities are concerned about the lack of scientific evidence on HRT from randomized controlled trials. To help answer some of the concerns, they undertook one of the biggest research programs ever, the Women's Health Initiative. This study involved 27,500 women in the HRT evaluation, 48,000 in a dietary modification evaluation, 45,000 in an evaluation of calcium and vitamin D, and 100,000 in an observational trial. Recruitment of the sample will finish in 1998 and the women will be followed for up to 9 years.

Now Versus the Future

Women who start taking HRT in their 50s, with the intention of using it long term for the prevention of ill health in older age, are looking to reap the benefits of their decision in up to 30 years' time. Will the balance between risks and benefits still be the same in the year 2020 as they are now? The answer to this question is "almost certainly not."

The number of people dying of heart disease in the United States, Australia, and other developed countries is gradually decreasing. If this decrease continues for the next 30 years as it has done for the past 20 years or so, then women who are currently in their 40s and 50s will have a lower chance of dying of heart disease than will women currently in their 70s and 80s, whether the younger group takes HRT or not. It is likely that HRT will help to make that chance lower still. However, whereas heart disease is declining, breast cancer is unfortunately becoming more common. So, although heart disease is a much more common disease than breast cancer at the moment, by the time the current generation of women taking HRT reach older age, the gap will have narrowed. This raises a serious question: Will HRT cause more disease and death than it prevents?

Living Longer Versus Feeling Well Now

So far, the discussion of the risks and benefits of HRT has been in relation to major illness and death because this is the primary interest of many researchers. However, most women are also concerned about how they feel day to day. For healthy women taking HRT long term, in pursuit of a longer life or healthier old age, how HRT affects them in the short term may well influence whether they continue with the therapy. For women who have side effects of the therapy, it may become a trade-off between how well they feel now and how well they may be when they are older.

The information available on the effects of HRT on the day-to-day health and well-being of women is limited. Although the therapy is promoted as maintaining the elasticity and "youth" of skin, there is remarkably little actual research that backs this up. Similarly, there is little evidence of an effect of HRT on moods, energy levels, and well-being. This does not necessarily mean that these benefits do not exist, because very few studies have even looked for them. However, it does mean that they are not proven effects of HRT.

Certainly, many women dislike the continuation or renewal of monthly menstrual bleeding that accompanies many forms of HRT.

Also, it is known that a small proportion of women who take HRT have unexplained or irregular bleeding while using the hormones (Archer et al. 1994). As well as causing some discomfort and distress, this may result in additional visits to the doctor and changes of prescription to find the right hormones and the right doses for each individual woman. For some women, unexpected bleeding will need to be investigated further, requiring tests and exploratory procedures. A small group of these women will have a hysterectomy as a result of their use of HRT.

Other side effects of HRT are similar to those of the pill and are often linked to the progestin component of the therapy. They include weight gain, headaches, and moodiness or depression. An increase in the risk of gallbladder disease is a known consequence of long-term use of HRT ; more women taking HRT have their gallbladder removed than do women who do not use the treatment (Petitti et al. 1988).

Weighing the Health Effects of Long-Term Use

If we put all this together, the picture regarding the long-term use of HRT starts to look less healthy. The benefits may not be as great as has been claimed, and the risks may be greater. The assessments of benefits and risks usually do not take into account other factors that are of great importance to women, such as how they feel day to day while taking HRT, whether they continue to have periods, and the fact that they may need a greater number of medical checks and tests. The conditions for which long-term use of HRT is recommended may be less common anyway, and the ones it might cause may affect more women. Amid all this uncertainty—all the "it may, but it might not"—caution is the only safe path.

After all, the lessons of the past few decades tell us that the promises for new drugs and therapies are often overly glossy and that a measure of skepticism and caution is appropriate. Within the past few decades, women have been promised so much by pharmaceutical companies and have experienced some major problems as well as the benefits. Experience has taught us that it is rare for good to come from new drugs or new products without there also being risks attached—which often do not appear until much later. Examples are the intrauterine device, silicon breast implants, the oral contraceptive pill, and human pituitary gonadotropin and other fertility drugs. Thus, healthy skepticism may not be out of place. As with so many other treatments before HRT, it is worth remembering that HRT is being increasingly prescribed for healthy women.

Even HRT itself already has one cloud over its head. Originally, just estrogen was used for the relief of hot flashes. However, a large increase in the occurrence of cancer of the endometrium (the lining of the uterus) among women using estrogen in the United States made clinicians and researchers aware that it can be unsafe for women to take estrogen for long periods of time. To counter this problem, progestin is usually now prescribed together with estrogen for women who have a uterus to counteract the effects of estrogen on the endometrium. The current evidence suggests that this combined treatment may not carry any increased risk of endometrial cancer (Weiss and Hill 1996).

It took around 25 years for the cancer-causing potential of estrogen used on its own to become apparent, and it took a further 3 years for its use to decline in response to research findings about the cancer link. Yet currently women are again being encouraged to embrace long-term use of hormone therapy for disease prevention before conclusive evidence of benefits and risks are established.

The Social Agenda

Even if we accept for the time being that the scientific claims for HRT turn out to be true, is this the only reason HRT is being so heavily promoted? Consider for a moment what menopause signifies to women and to society in general. Menopause signifies the end of a woman's reproductive life. Stereotypes that are prevalent in Western societies such as ours characterize the menopausal and aging woman very negatively, with concepts ranging from "unattractive" and "possibly slightly deranged" to "a burden on society." As a society, we fear old age and death. We do not value our elderly. We do not consider them wise or experienced or having much to offer, but rather as a burden and an increasing drain on an overstretched health and welfare budget. For women, menopause is a very clear marker of the aging process, and one for which there is no direct equivalent for men.

Is it possible, then, that the promotion of HRT is a consequence of this fear of aging? After all, by taking HRT from the start of the menopause and continuing to take it, women can effectively postpone menopause. By denying menopause and the aging process that it signifies, we are also reinforcing the view that women are valuable to society only when they are young, physically attractive, and able to bear children. Maybe it is this view of women that leads men to view menopause as catastrophic, whereas women are more inclined to consider it a natural developmental process.

In the meantime, there is another concerning aspect of the promotion of the use of HRT. Many women are choosing not to take HRT, whereas other women's circumstances prevent them from undergoing long-term treatment. These women include those who choose to be cautious, those who do not like the idea of being medicated for the remainder of their lives, those whose family or personal medical histories throw some doubt over the benefit of HRT for them, those who have taken the therapy and have experienced unacceptable side effects, and those who are unwilling to accept the cost and increased degree of medical surveillance that frequently accompanies HRT prescription from cautious doctors. There is the possibility that women who choose not to take HRT may be made to feel responsible should ill health occur. If they break a hip in old age or suffer from heart disease, who will they have to blame but themselves? If they had only taken their pills or stuck to their patches, this would not have happened. They are being warned that they will increase the burden that old women represent in an aging society that does not value its elderly. We are all aware of women's tendency to accept blame and to feel guilt.

Some of the promotion of HRT surreptitiously plays on women's fears. To encourage women to take preventive action against ill health at older ages by using HRT, women have been made aware of the conditions that may affect them. Women have been "frightened" into taking action. The linking of heart disease and osteoporosis with menopause—so that menopause, rather than the aging process itself, is seen as a cause of these diseases—allows HRT to become the focus of preventive approaches.

Although this development may have some advantages for women, it also has the potential disadvantage of making ill health and old age seem to be the necessary consequences of menopause. Other approaches to maintaining health and preventing disease are not receiving the attention that HRT receives and so do not appear as real alternatives to many women, whereas the importance of building health earlier in their lives has been neglected.

Summary

The question to be answered about HRT is not whether it offers benefits to women—it clearly does—but whether the risks it presents outweigh those benefits. Consider the uncertainties and gaps in the scientific evidence about the value and the risks of HRT and the social impact of helping to reinforce the negative view of older women in our society. Are we still sure that HRT is a major breakthrough that will safeguard women's health into older age?

References

Archer DF, Pickar JH, Bottiglioni F, et al: Bleeding patterns in postmenopausal women taking continuous combined or sequential regimens of conjugated estrogens with medroxyprogesterone acetate. Obstetrics and Gynecology 83:686–692, 1994

Barrett-Connor E: Postmenopausal estrogen and prevention bias. Annals of Internal Medicine 115:455–456, 1991

Barrett-Connor E: Postmenopausal estrogen and the risk of breast cancer. Annals of Epidemiology 4:177–180, 1994

Barrett-Connor E: The menopause, hormone replacement, and cardiovascular disease: the epidemiologic evidence. Maturitas 23:225–232, 1996

Grady D, Rubin SM, Petitti DB, et al: Hormone therapy to prevent disease and prolong life in postmenopausal women. Annals of Internal Medicine 117:1016–1037, 1992

Petitti DB: Coronary heart disease and estrogen replacement therapy: can compliance bias explain the results of observational studies? Annals of Epidemiology 4:115–118, 1994

Petitti DB, Sidney S, Periman JA: Increased risk of cholecystectomy in users of supplemental estrogen. Gastroenterology 94:91–95, 1988

Stampfer MJ, Colditz GA: Estrogen replacement and coronary heart disease: a quantitative assessment of the epidemiologic evidence. Preventive Medicine 20:47–63, 1991

Steinberg KK, Thacker SB, Smith SJ, et al: A meta-analysis of the effect of estrogen replacement therapy on the risk of breast cancer. Journal of the American Medical Association 265:1985–1990, 1991

Wark JD: Osteoporotic fractures: background and prevention strategies. Maturitas 23:191–206, 1996

Weiss NS, Hill DA: Postmenopausal estrogens and progestogens and the incidence of gynecologic cancer. Maturitas 23:233–238, 1996

CHAPTER 6

Consumers or Victims? The Menopause, Hormone Therapy, and the Mass Media

Ann Westmore

The debate about the appropriate place in women's lives of menopause-related hormone therapy has given rise to extensive mass media coverage since the late 1950s. The coverage has tended to characterize menopause and the use of hormone therapy in two divergent ways. On the one hand, much popular opinion and many medical experts have portrayed the menopause as a major negative life event, of the same magnitude as the loss of a spouse or a job. The U.S. Congress Office of Technology Assessment (1992) has summarized the situation as follows:

> Menopause has come to signify the end of reproduction and the acceleration of aging, both of which are viewed with dread by

> many members of Western societies that extol the family and youthful sexuality. (p. 14)

The stereotypical image, repeated consistently in the print media and the medical press, is that women experiencing the menopause are unhappy people whose lives can be restored by becoming consumers of hormones. In contrast, menopause is also portrayed as a normal—though sometimes difficult and often misunderstood—part of life for women. Those who share this view tend to regard hormone replacement therapy (HRT) as a treatment prescribed too readily by some doctors and without adequate discussion of the nondrug alternatives and risks. The Australian feminist author Germaine Greer, a self-acknowledged skeptic of the newfound interest of the medical profession and pharmaceutical industry in women past childbearing age, has put it this way (Greer 1991):

> Women's happiness consists, it seems, in becoming a more exact fit to a man. Just as the definitions of sexual intercourse current in the later twentieth century sought to confer upon women an orgasm as much like a man's as possible, now a woman's aging pattern is meant to keep step (pp. 208–209).

Women who struggle to emulate men can be seen as victims of powerful commercial, professional, and paternalistic interests whose objective is to sell an impossible dream. The debate shows every sign of continuing and gives rise to questions such as "Who or what is driving the debate about hormone therapy during menopause and the years following it?" "To what extent is the hormone technology in control of its own destiny, and to what extent can that destiny be shaped by human agency?"

Highs and Lows of Hormone Therapy

Mass-circulation books and relevant articles in women's magazines and newspapers are a productive place to start examining these questions (Westmore 1995). From the late 1950s to the mid-1970s, estrogen was promoted as the way to become *Feminine Forever* (Wilson 1966) and to achieve a state of *No Change* (Cooper 1975). For those with lingering doubts, articles like "Menopause: Is There a Cure?" (Davidson 1968) suggested that there were many benefits and some ill-defined risks to be considered. Almost without exception during this era, menopause was characterized in the mass media as a hateful time for women as well as for their families and business colleagues. Menopause was also commonly portrayed as a serious hormone deficiency disease, affecting most if not all women, that was "curable" with estrogen. The media accepted virtually without question the notion that the levels of sex hormones of women in their prime reproductive years (20s and 30s) were desirable for women in their later years. Another issue that did not receive much attention was the inevitable bias inherent in short-term research findings and in research based on self-selected groups of women seeking treatment in the health care system.

From late 1975 to the early 1980s, the reputation of adjuvant estrogen as an aid to older women plummeted. The first alarm bells sounded with publication of reports in December 1975 by two groups of U.S. scientists who independently concluded that women with an intact uterus who took estrogen for several years were significantly more likely to develop endometrial cancer than those not taking the hormone. With these and later reports of an association, troubling headlines like "Hormones and Cancer: Is There a Connection?" (Nourse 1976) found their way into women's magazines. Pharmaceutical advertisements for hormone therapies faded from sight and a more cautious approach to estrogen use emerged, resulting in a rapid drop in sales of the hormone. This was followed by a decline in the incidence of endometrial cancer.

There are numerous instances in which sales of pharmaceutical products have crashed after research has revealed a link with a major health problem, thalidomide being a case in point. Not so estrogen. The reason it escaped this fate was that pharmaceutical companies and medical scientists studying the undesirable effect of estrogen on the endometrium found a way to provide protection against endometrial cancer. This involved prescribing progestin (a manufactured version of the sex hormone progesterone) on all or some days of estrogen use. However, a downside to combining progestin with estrogen soon emerged. The combination was frequently associated with unpleasant side effects, both physical (breast tenderness, bloating, expected or unexpected bleeding, weight gain) and psychological (anxiety, depression, irritability). To this day these symptoms have proved sufficiently disturbing to persuade many women who start on hormone therapy to come off it within a year or two.

From the 1980s on, the combination of estrogen and progestin was widely proclaimed as a safe way to reverse the hormone deficiency said to start around the time of menopause, as well as to achieve good health, good looks, and a happy disposition. Some studies suggested that hormone therapy alleviated acute symptoms of menopause—for instance, hot flashes and vaginal dryness—and averted major long-term causes of ill health and poor quality of life in women, particularly heart disease and osteoporosis. Newspapers and magazines announced that hormone therapy was back in favor, with articles bearing headlines such as "Pills' Flush of Success Takes the Heat Out of Life" (Stewart 1993) and "The Good News About Osteoporosis" (Turner 1990).

The alarm bells have been ringing again recently with the suggestion that hormone therapy used for 5 years or longer significantly increases the likelihood of breast cancer and other unwanted sequelae, including hysterectomy (U.S. Congress Office of Technology Assessment 1992). Although conclusive studies examining a possible link between hormone use and breast cancer will not be available for some years, the mass media coverage has reverted to cautious mode, with a renewed emphasis on the importance of examining risks as well as benefits before embarking on hormone therapy (Bell 1991; Farrell and Westmore 1993; Finkel 1993; Westmore 1992).

A significant recent development in the medical press is the advent of thoughtful questioning of the assertion that the estrogen levels of most menopausal women are deficient. As stated by Rosenberg (1993), this line of argument can be sustained only if there is a sound reason to focus entirely on the occurrence of hot flashes, urogenital changes, fractures, and heart disease as the health problems of most concern to older women. Once the focus is shifted to other major health problems experienced by older women, such as cancers of the breast, endometrium, and ovaries, together with fibroids and endometriosis, then it can just as well be argued that postmenopausal women produce a more desirable level of estrogen for their life stage than their premenopausal sisters (Rosenberg 1993). The reasons for regarding the estrogen levels of the fertile years, rather than the estrogen levels of, say, childhood or the postmenopause, as the physiological norm have never been explained satisfactorily. After all, women in developed countries are fertile for fewer than 30 years of their lifetimes on average, and during the other 50 or so years they are neither ovulating nor menstruating. According to this reasoning, it is the high estrogen levels during the reproductive years that are anomalous.

Hormone Therapy as a Newsworthy Topic

The newsworthiness of menopause-related hormone therapy has been demonstrated over many years by the extensive media coverage it has received. One view is that this reflects the intrinsic need of most women for hormonal support because "post-menopause is a potential 'hormone deficiency disease'" (Cabot 1991, p. 18). An alternative explanation is that the newsworthiness of menopause is a direct result of publicity that is generated and funded by those pharmaceutical companies that have a vested interest in seeing it accepted and used by women throughout the last third of their lives (Coney 1991). Whether the community accepts one of these viewpoints or some other, the place of hormone therapy in women's lives will depend to some extent on the media's ability to accurately present the claims for and against these divergent views, expose underlying assumptions, and provide space and air time to enable scrutiny of them.

There is no obvious reason why this should not occur in countries like the United States and Australia, because decisions to publish or broadcast stories are made in a social and cultural setting that is mercifully free of censorship. These decisions rely on interchanges among editors, producers, presenters, journalists, and/or media proprietors who make judgments about newsworthiness according to their own tastes and values and those of other people whose views they respect—family members, friends, colleagues, competitors, and business acquaintances, for instance.

Focusing on this human input serves as a reminder that the news is not an independent, autonomous entity but a human construct, a set of conventions that makes sense in a given time and place. Because what is considered newsworthy is liable to change as ideas and values alter, what constitutes "news" is rightly a subject for debate. Thus, if society regards menopause as a purely biological phenomenon—a design fault of female biology—then it may expect chemicals such as hormones to provide the "solution." However, if menopause is considered to have social, economic, and political components in addition to a contribution from biology, then what constitutes news about it becomes much broader. For example, social policies and non-drug approaches to improving quality of life and health in older women become just as relevant as information on hormones.

Opportunities to Reinforce or Upturn Prevailing Views

To say that the mass media reflects prevailing attitudes is to imply a sameness of outlook and behavior within media outlets and to neglect the diversity of attitudes and approaches, even within a single print media or broadcasting body.

The Selection of Experts

The multicultural nature of media organizations in many countries provides an opening for a variety of attitudes, preferences, choices, and decisions, for example, in the matter of selecting "experts" who provide information and advice on subjects about which journalists have limited knowledge or skills. Medical and scientific experts are especially useful to the media not just because of their special knowledge but because they are regarded as having abundant credibility and authority. This is because they have traditionally embodied the values of objectivity and disinterested searching for truth (Nelkin 1987).

From the 1950s to the early 1980s, the experts about menopause and hormone treatments typically quoted in the mass media were gynecologists and endocrinologists. The voices of women consumers and patients, nonmedical therapists, and consumer health advocates were notably absent. Family doctors who saw a broad cross-section of women were not regarded as having expertise on the subject and their views were not heard, nor were those of other sorts of medical specialists—for instance, those working in cancer management who may have had something relevant to say. Recognition of expertise about menopause in this era required an understanding of women's reproductive organs and associated hormonal influences.

These days, articles and programs about menopause carry the views of a more diverse selection of experts, including consumer health representatives, epidemiologists, cancer specialists, sociologists and anthropologists who have talked to women experiencing menopause or postmenopause, historians of science, economists, and a range of nonmedical and medical practitioners in the health care area. This change has occurred not by chance but because of activity on several fronts.

Critics of the medical model of menopause exposed its inability to explain why women from different cultures, as well as many women in developed societies, have a far more positive experience of menopause than suggested by the model. In addition, many previously underrepresented groups took a lead from the consumer health movement and argued that they, too, had relevant expertise.

The medical profession's claim to objectivity about hormone therapy also came under challenge, based on its close links with the pharmaceutical industry. Most people accept that pharmaceutical companies can play an important role in health care. But it is also apparent that medical judgments may be unduly influenced by the closeness of medicine's ties with the industry, as exemplified by its funding of medical research studies, sponsorship of medical conferences and dinners, and financial assistance to fund patient education materials. Senior members of the medical profession have argued for the introduction of stronger safeguards to ensure that pharmaceutical industry funding does not compromise the education of doctors and the care and education of patients (Moulds 1993).

Choice of Words and Images

The tools of trade of journalists—words and images—are inevitably charged with meaning and subtlety. Depending on which choices are made, vastly different impressions are conveyed to audiences. The selection and content of stories and broadcasts can never be neutral, nor is this desirable. However, the onus is on journalists to present issues and analyses clearly and, where controversy exists, to air different points of view. The extent to which competing arguments are presented in the mass media has been a subject of considerable soul-searching by many journalists.

An existing code of journalistic ethics calls on journalists to "report and interpret the news with scrupulous honesty by striving to disclose all essential facts and by not suppressing relevant, available facts or by distorting by wrong or improper emphasis" (Media Entertainment and Arts Alliance 1993, p. 5). In reviewing the code, journalists are asking themselves if meeting this test requires that they offer a person an opportunity to respond to unfavorable material in the same item that discloses it (Media Entertainment and Arts Alliance 1993).

Reliance on "Old" News

The mass media has a voracious appetite for entertainment and information, and satisfying this hunger is a major part of any journalist's work. Tight time deadlines, space limitations, and a journalist's lack of knowledge about a particular subject inevitably lead to overreliance on previously published or broadcast information. The tone and assumptions of previous reports tend to be picked up and carried forward to a new audience (Henningham 1990).

Effect of the "Youth Factor"

Another influence on the tone and content of media coverage of issues like menopause and hormone therapy relates to the "youth factor," the tendency for print and broadcast journalism to be a young person's occupation. Although youthfulness as such does not in any way preclude an interest in aging processes, including menopause, it has been found that attitudes to menopause shift as experience takes over from expectation. That is, as women experience menopause, their feelings about it tend to become more positive (Avis and McKinlay 1991). It follows that if coverage of menopause is handled mainly by the young, the picture ultimately presented in the mass media may be unduly pessimistic, and the prospect of a technological "cure" in the form of hormone formulations may receive undue prominence.

Summary

The mass media is an infinitely diverse and amorphous forum in which complex social interactions, considered choices, personal experiences, and scientific information meet. An understanding of the forces at work in the setting of the newspaper office, radio station, or television studio has the potential to empower women to reshape the debate about menopause and hormone therapy and to discard the stereotypes of consumer and victim.

References

Avis NE, McKinlay SM: A longitudinal analysis of women's attitudes toward the menopause: results from the Massachusetts Women's Health Study. Maturitas 13:65–79, 1991

Bell G: The selling of HRT. The Bulletin, July 30, 1991

Cabot S: Menopause: you can give it a miss. Sydney, New South Wales Women's Health Advisory Service, 1991
Coney S: The Menopause Industry. Auckland, New Zealand, Penguin Books, 1991
Cooper W: No Change: A Biological Revolution for Women. Arrow Books, 1975
Davidson B: Menopause: is there a cure? New Idea, March 10, 1968
Farrell E, Westmore A: The HRT Handbook. Melbourne, Anne O'Donovan, 1993
Finkel E: The great hormone balancing act. The Age, April 21, 1993
Greer G: The Change. London, Hamish Hamilton, 1991
Henningham J (ed): Issues in Australian Journalism. Melbourne, Longman Cheshire, 1990, p 31
Media, Entertainment and Arts Alliance (Australia): Ethics Review Committee Issues Paper (unpublished). Sydney, Media, Entertainment and Arts Alliance, December 1993
Moulds R: Promoting and advertising therapeutic goods. Medical Journal of Australia 157:513–514, 1993
Nelkin D: Controversies and the authority of science, in Scientific Controversies. Edited by Engelhardt HT, Caplan AL. London, Cambridge University Press, 1987, pp 283–293
Nourse A: Hormones and cancer: is there a connection? Woman's Day, February 1976
Rosenberg L: Hormone replacement therapy: the need for reconsideration. American Journal of Public Health 83:1670–1673, 1993
Stewart M: Pills' flush of success takes the heat out of life. The Age, April 21, 1993
Turner B: The good news about osteoporosis. Ita, August 1990
U.S. Congress Office of Technology Assessment: The Menopause, Hormone Therapy and Women's Health. Washington, DC, Government Printing Office, 1992
Westmore A: Long-term HRT use questioned. Australian Doctor, October 9, 1992
Westmore A: Appropriation of value-laden concepts in the menopause/hormone replacement therapy co-construction. Master of Science Thesis, University of Melbourne, 1995
Wilson R: Feminine Forever. London, WH Allen, 1966

CHAPTER 7

Psychosocial Aspects of Menopause

Malkah T. Notman

The onset of menopause has been a subject of a great many stereotypes and of mythology and prejudice. In the past 10 years or so, there has been an accumulating body of research, evidence, and personal accounts that document that these expectations are not necessarily true—that menopause varies considerably with each woman and her life situation and with the culture in which she lives, and that many of the symptoms that were thought to accompany menopause are not universal. Even those that are quite common in developed countries are not necessarily as common in other places. Perhaps even the biology of menopause varies (Lock 1995).

In the 1960s there was also the concept that estrogen would maintain a woman's femininity. This was based on the belief that a woman's femininity was linked to her reproductive capacity.

Femininity is a very complicated concept. We now understand it to be a variable set of expectations that are part of what we now call *gender role.* This consists of attitudes and behaviors that are expected of a woman within a particular culture. Even though these are very broad and poorly defined, there are prevailing ideas about what being feminine means, and they vary at different times in history and in different places. There is also a pejorative aspect to being considered "unfeminine." Someone who is considered unfeminine is regarded critically. Nevertheless, the idea that one could stay feminine forever if one replaced the "lost" hormones was part of the concept that a woman's femininity is linked to her youth and to her reproductive life, rather than more generally based on qualities of personality or behavior that also change during the life cycle. The idea that femininity was dependent on estrogens led doctors and women to think that replacement hormones would be an important factor in preserving what was considered an essential quality for women. Actually, replacement hormones do not sustain reproduction or prolong youth, so if they are taken, it must be for other reasons.

There has also been confusion between which changes derive from the menopause itself and which are really part of normal aging. Because the menopause represents a transition that is part of getting older, it is also seen as a symbol of aging. This is not usually a positive sign. In some cultures, women do not have access to effective contraception and continue to bear children until the menopause. They can feel relieved when fertility ends and they can stop childbearing. For example, Mayan women in Valladolid, Mexico, who have multiple pregnancies, often with complications, looked forward to their menopause (Beyene 1989). These women did not complain of any menopausal symptoms, not even hot flashes, which are reported in about two-thirds of women in most industrialized societies. The anthropologists who studied the women in Mexico also compared their experiences with those of villagers in Stira, Greece. The Greek women also reported menopause as the beginning of a period of freedom from restrictions and activities and relief at not bearing children, but they also strongly associated menopause with the undesirable status of growing old. Seventy-five percent of these Greek women did report hot flashes even though they considered menopause to be a natural state. However, they did not seek medical attention for these symptoms.

Aging is not a positive experience in most cultures. Because childbearing may end long before menopause if contraception is available, if menopause is regarded primarily as a sign of aging, it can precipitate distress about growing older. Sexual attractiveness is also associated with youth, and an older woman feels less valued and less attractive. She is often concerned about how young she looks and how she is regarded. When a woman's status is closely connected with being able to bear children, the loss of this role of being a valuable woman can then be very important. In a society where there are no options for women except for family roles, menopause can be more distressing and women can feel this role loss intensely. Other possibilities, such as paid work outside the home or being able to participate in a wider range of valued community activities, are important when they reach this phase. This observation is supported by studies linking menopausal symptomatology and social class. Middle- and upper-class women have described less symptomatology than those with more constraints in their lives (see Chapter 2).

However, it is important to recognize that these feelings are not inevitably or inherently part of the menopause itself, but rather are related to life transitions and how these transitions are regarded and valued. It is also necessary to distinguish feelings that are due to family stresses and changes, marital problems, difficulties with children, and concerns about aging from menopausal symptoms. Responses that are primarily part of life cycle developments also do not respond to hormone replacement.

Feminist Critique

Feminist writing has voiced some opposition to hormone replacement therapy (HRT). This opposition has a number of sources, including distrust of the medical establishment in other areas as well. Some have the view that the medical profession tends to take over what might be considered a natural event, such as childbirth, as well as the menopause. The mistrust of the medical establishment has complex roots, but it is also based on the fact that, until recently, most doctors have been males. The power differential between the male doctor and the female patient has thus played a role. In the early part of the century, medicine was also more paternalistic: the doctor was the authority who told the patient what to do and did not usually involve the patient in any collaborative decision making. This dynamic was accentuated by the societal power differences between males and females. There are many examples in recent history where women patients and research subjects were not given adequate data, with disastrous results. The diethylstilbestrol (DES) tragedy is an example. In the 1960s, many women were given DES as a way of forestalling possible threatened miscarriages. It later turned out that DES has a harmful effect on the baby, with many problems later in life, including infertility, cancer, and other defects. As discussed in Chapter 5, the recent problems with intrauterine devices are examples of situations in which the medical establishment either did not have adequate data or did not reveal the data to those at risk or those who believed they had experienced problems. As the information about damaging effects emerged, suspicions about medical advice and information increased.

Another important determinant of a woman's reaction to menopause is her identification with her mother. If her mother had a difficult menopause or suffered from depression or symptoms in her middle years, a woman can associate this with menopause and feel that this is what she must expect as well.

Sexuality

Population-based data reported in Chapter 2 (Dennerstein et al. 1994) indicate that some women experience a decline in sexual functioning with the menopausal transition. This can be difficult to interpret, because male partners can be less interested, or women can expect to be less sexual as they grow older. Postmenopausal vaginal dryness can also create dyspareunia. Hot flashes can feel as if a woman's sexual status is being exposed and can feel very embarrassing. Family stresses and sexual changes may well be part of a woman's middle years, and the menopause can be blamed for these problems.

For a woman who reaches the menopausal period, children may be either adolescents and difficult to manage or older and embarking on their own marriages and their new lives. A woman who is concerned about her attractiveness or her sexual desirability can find the competitive aspects of her relationship with a young, attractive daughter difficult. She can feel displaced, envious, and displeased with her life, even though she also loves her daughter and wants the best for her. In fact, some women who are not yet menopausal find themselves pregnant just at the time that their daughter is getting married or going off with her own relationship. They may not be aware of these competitive feelings but may unconsciously act on them.

Midlife sexual changes that occur in both women and men can also create problems. One of the physical changes that accompanies menopause is diminished vaginal lubrication, and as a result a woman can be slower to respond sexually. A man may need increased time to become aroused and longer time between periods of arousal, and there may be delay in ejaculation. If the man is distressed by these changes in himself, he can blame his partner and withdraw from her for not being responsive or exciting enough. Sometimes the man's midlife reassessment period also involves becoming aware of other disappointments and frustrations, and sometimes he blames them on his marriage. A man who breaks up a marriage in midlife may be leaving a wife who is menopausal. Frequently he goes off with a younger woman. This is difficult whenever it happens, but if it occurs at a time of her menopause, the woman can blame herself for the loss of the marriage. She may feel that the changes in her sexual response are truly "the problem" and that this is an important element in her husband's disappointment.

HRT does help vaginal dryness. Both oral estrogen and vaginal creams improve lubrication. It is possible to treat these symptoms with lubricants that are not hormonal, but many women do take estrogen for these symptoms. Some women feel that the self-confidence they gain from their more predictable response also helps diminish sexual anxiety.

Mood, Cognitive Functioning, and Psychological Aspects

A population-based, follow-up study (Dennerstein et al 1997) described in Chapter 2 indicated that women's moods tend to be lowered in the 2 years following the final menstrual period. Mood then improves spontaneously. But depression is not intrinsically part of the menopausal experience. It used to be said that menopause is inevitably associated with distress and depression; this has been shown by many studies not to be the case. An individual woman may, however, feel depressed because of her own association of the menopause with an undesirable state of life and its problems.

Some studies (e.g., Sherwin and Phillips 1990) suggest that, for women who have had a hysterectomy, replacement estrogen has some effect on mood. This is still very controversial, and it is important to recognize that estrogens are not effective in treating clinical depression generally, although a recent study suggests that high-dose estrogen patches may be effective for postpartum depression (Gregoire et al. 1996).

Some recent literature (van Duijn 1997) suggests that women who take HRT are spared some of the cognitive impairment of Alzheimer's disease and aging. This is also not conclusive and is not an adequate indication for HRT. Estrogens are also not effective treatments for panic disorders or emotional symptoms and disorders.

To understand the psychological changes of the menopause, it is important to consider the whole reproductive time clock within which women live and make choices. Although a particular woman may not have children because of circumstances or her own wishes, many women grow up believing—positively or negatively—that childbearing is part of their expectation of life. For most women, this represents a positive part of reaching adulthood and an identification with their mothers and women in general.

The girl at menarche is told that she will have periods until menopause and that she can get pregnant until then. This may be something she feels positively about, or it may feel like a risk she runs. Being told that she can become pregnant can be perceived as a warning or a danger. For most young girls, menopause does not seem to be a concrete reality or something to think about until much later. When a woman reaches her late 20s and early 30s, it is very much more in the background as a potential ending of her possibilities for having children and begins to exert its influence on her choices about marriage and work.

This is a different sense of urgency than exists for men, who can make choices without this biological deadline hanging over their heads. Women are thus likely to think about the menopause and the finiteness of their reproductive years much earlier than the time of the actual menopause, which is at about age 50. For many women who have access to contraception, the ending of their actual childbearing occurs many years before menopause. It is important to recognize this in sorting out the psychological experience of the menopause itself, because the feelings about ending childbearing do not necessarily occur at the time of the menopause. Menopause acquires an additional immediacy for women who start their childbearing late. In these situations, however, concern about fertility does not coincide with the actual menopausal time but precedes it. The new reproductive technologies can extend the fertile period, although they are expensive and not available to everyone.

For many women, menopause is thus not a highly significant event in itself. A Massachusetts study (McKinlay and McKinlay 1987) of women of menopausal age indicated that there are more concerns as women approach menopause than during it or afterward and that the vast majority of women do not seek health care more often around this time. Some report relief, regret at missed opportunities, or distress at aging or a variety of individual experiences and meanings. These will not be addressed by HRT but can be helped by support, education, and, if needed, psychotherapy.

There has been a change in the time during which women expect to be bearing children in Western industrialized societies. From the dictum of an earlier period that stated "have your first child before the age of 30," the medical advice has shifted. As women's health has improved, later childbearing has become less risky and many women have invested in work and careers before they marry. The age at first pregnancy varies from teenagers, who constitute a large group of women having a first pregnancy, to women who are having their first babies in their late 30s and early 40s. There is currently some concern about infertility, which appears to be greater in women waiting until they are older when they begin having children.

Summary

We do not have norms of what normal life should be like psychologically for the postmenopausal years. Neither have we conceptualized what is normal for women in this postparental period. In recent years, with increasing work opportunities for women and also the economic necessity for many women to work, it is clear that the ending of childbearing is accompanied by a shift in women's development and activities. There are many possibilities for expansion and for personal growth. Some of the early models conceptualizing menopause primarily in terms of loss, mourning, and regret need to be revised to reflect these changes in opportunities, social conditions, life expectancy, and our greater knowledge about women's lives.

References

Beyene Y: From Menarche to Menopause. New York, SUNY Press, 1989
Dennerstein L, Smith AMA, Morse CA, et al: Sexuality and the Menopause. Journal of Psychosomatic Obstetrics and Gynaecology 15:59–66, 1994

Dennerstein L, Dudley E, Burger H: Wellbeing and the menopausal transition. Journal of Psychosomatic Obstetrics and Gynaecology 18:95–101, 1997

Gregoire AJP, Kumar R, Everitt B, et al: Transdermal oestrogen for treatment of severe postnatal depression. Lancet 347(9006):930–933, 1996

Lock M: Women, middle age and menopause in Japan and North America. NASPO Annual Meeting Abstracts. Womens Health Issues 5(2):74, 1995

McKinlay S, McKinlay J: Health status and behavior associated with menopause. American Journal of Epidemiology 125:110–121, 1987

Sherwin B, Phillips S: Estrogen and cognitive functioning in surgically menopausal women, in Multidisciplinary Perspectives on Menopause. Edited by Flint M, Kronenberg F, Utian W. Annals of the New York Academy of Sciences 592:474–475, 1990

van Duijn CM: Menopause and the brain. Journal of Psychosomatic Obstetrics and Gynaecology 18:121–125, 1997

CHAPTER 8

The Role of Exercise and Diet in Midlife Health

Janet Guthrie

Almost every time you pick up a pamphlet or publication on menopause, you see the two words *exercise* and *diet*. Either the authors are recommending that you improve these lifestyle variables to maintain good health, or they are suggesting that lack of exercise and poor diet may contribute to health problems and menopausal symptoms.

Appropriate lifestyle factors, in particular exercise and diet, may be of benefit in maintaining health and well-being in the face of physiological and psychosocial stressors. The aim of this chapter is to explain what is meant by diet and exercise and their importance in midlife health and to try to quantify these two variables: that is, what "prescription" can be given to midlife women with regard to their exercise and diet for the maintenance of good health during and after this midlife period?

Exercise and diet are not suggested as alternatives to hormone replacement therapy (HRT), but they are necessary additions to HRT and are essential for enhancing long-term health. In some cases they may even eliminate the need for HRT.

Physical activity—that is, the bodily exertion of energy—is probably a better term for our purposes than *exercise.* Similarly, the word *nutrition* is preferable to the word *diet*: we shall be looking at certain nutrients that should be included or eliminated from the diet rather than an overall dietary plan. Nutrition and its importance in relation to the blood fat profile and bone density are discussed.

The health problems that are associated with the reduction in ovarian function and for which physical activity and diet may provide some help fall broadly into four categories: 1) diseases of the heart and blood vessels (cardiovascular disease), 2) osteoporosis, 3) vaginal and urinary tract disorders (genitourinary problems), and 4) hot flashes and sweats.

Risk Factors for Cardiovascular Disease

Risk factors are aspects of a woman's lifestyle, physical condition, and medical history that can increase her chances of developing certain health disorders. If she has more than one risk factor, it is not just a case of adding them up, but of multiplying them. That is, having more than one risk factor for heart disease greatly increases the risk of having a heart attack. A family history of cardiovascular disease or a known abnormal finding, such as a heart murmur, on a physical exam are examples of medical history risk factors. The risk factors for heart disease and stroke include high blood fats (plasma lipids) such as cholesterol, high blood pressure, smoking, and obesity and are related to lifestyle factors.

Plasma Lipids

Cholesterol travels in the blood in the form of lipoproteins, that is, a combination of fat and protein. There are two main fractions of lipoproteins in the blood: the low-density lipoproteins (LDLs) and the high-density lipoproteins (HDLs). HDLs are the "good" fraction and LDLs are the "bad" fraction. In other words, the increased risk of heart disease associated with high cholesterol levels is strongly affected by the relative amounts of HDL and LDL. High LDL levels are likely to result in disease, whereas high HDL levels provide protection against heart disease.

Physical activity has been identified as increasing the amount of HDL in the blood. Including unsaturated fat products in the diet, restricting saturated fats, and keeping a healthy body weight are effective in lowering LDL levels. Saturated fats are found in meat and dairy fats and in some vegetable fats such as coconut and palm oil, which are often used in commercially prepared foods such as cakes, biscuits, and pastries. Unsaturated fat products include fish and vegetable oils.

A decrease in estradiol production by the ovaries is associated with a decrease in HDL cholesterol. However, regular physical activity is associated with higher levels of HDL cholesterol and with maintaining levels at the time of the menopause. Modest increases in physical activity levels—for example, walking three times per week for 20 minutes—led to smaller decreases in HDL cholesterol levels in postmenopausal American women in one study (Owens et al. 1992). The type of activity needed to raise HDL levels appears to reflect some type of sport or recreational activity (Cauley et al. 1986). Thus, energy expenditure of moderate intensity has been shown to be related to higher levels of HDL cholesterol.

If a woman's blood fat levels are well outside the normal range, a more intensive physical activity campaign than that recommended above is prescribed: 4 months of fairly intensive activity, for example, running 10–15 miles per week; or 7 months of moderately intensive activity, for example, walking 30 miles per week (Notelovitz 1990). Although some women take up running in midlife or later, the second recommendation seems more feasible. Walking 30 miles a week is the equivalent of walking approximately 1.5–2 hours per day. At first, walking time can be gradually increased—to up to an hour per day three times a week, as outlined in Table 8–1.

If you have been a nonexerciser all your life, it is not too late to start. A health check with your doctor is advisable, especially if you

Table 8–1. Exercise plan—3 times per week

Week 1	20 minutes walking per day
Week 2	30 minutes walking per day
Week 3	40 minutes walking per day
Week 4	50 minutes walking per day
Routine	60 minutes walking per day

intend to do vigorous activity, such as jogging.

The mechanism of the effect of physical activity on plasma cholesterol levels is unknown. Estrogen therapy appears to be promising in reducing the risk of coronary heart disease (see also Chapters 4and 5), and 50% of this reduction is being attributed to plasma lipid changes. So if we can modify our plasma lipids by increasing our levels of physical activity, we are halfway to reducing our risk without the use of hormone therapy.

Blood Pressure

High blood pressure (hypertension) usually causes no immediate symptoms but poses a long-term problem because of the stress it places on the heart and blood vessels. Hypertension requires treatment with specific drugs, but the following physical activity findings are very relevant.

Light activity—for example, walking or gardening—or moderately intense activity—for example, playing tennis, bicycling, swimming, or dancing—performed regularly by American women age 50 and over was shown to be associated with lower blood pressure and a lower prevalence of hypertension in one study (Reaven et al. 1991). High-intensity activities, such as playing squash, running, or doing aerobic exercises were also associated with lower resting blood pressure values. However, there was no statistically significant difference between the blood pressures of the high- and low-intensity exercise groups (Reaven et al. 1991).

Physical activity of light to moderate intensity may be a particularly effective nonpharmacological method of lowering blood pressure. It seems to have an effect on blood pressure beyond its role in weight control, independent of age, alcohol consumption, and estrogen use. All these factors have an independent effect on blood pressure. Again, the exact mechanism by which physical activity may lower blood pressure is not known.

Obesity

Weight gain is a common occurrence in midlife. Changes in weight are related to changes in heart disease risk factors; that is, weight gain is significantly associated with increases in blood pressure and levels of LDL cholesterol. The Melbourne Women's Midlife Health Project (Dennerstein et al. 1994) found that over 3 years, women who were experiencing the menopausal transition gained an average of 2.2 kg (4.8 pounds) in weight. Women who remained premenopausal during these 3 years gained an average of 1.3 kg (2.9 pounds). (Weight findings from J. R. Guthrie, unpublished data, 1997.)

The percentage of body fat can be calculated by measuring skin fold thickness at various sites. There is now evidence that the higher is the index of waist-hip circumference, the greater is the risk of coronary heart disease. U.S. population studies have repeatedly shown that active people have a much lower body fat mass than do more sedentary members of the community (Wing et al. 1991). In addition to an increase in energy expenditure by an increase in physical activity, a reduction in energy intake may be necessary—in particular, a reduction in fat intake, because fat is a high-energy food containing approximately twice as many calories per gram as carbohydrates and proteins.

Other Risk Factors

Smoking. Smoking is bad for every aspect of health, in particular, the heart and blood vessels. Smokers who have trouble quitting should seek guidance from programs specifically designed to help this problem.

Fibrinogen. An independent cardiovascular risk factor is the level of fibrinogen in the blood. Fibrinogen is a plasma protein that is essential to the blood clotting process. Like all plasma components, it must be kept within its normal concentration range because at higher values it participates in both the formation of unwanted blood clots and abnormal deposits on blood vessel walls. Both of these events may cause cardiovascular disease. Studies of European women (Ernst 1993) have shown that regular, medium-intensity exercise—three times a week for approximately 60 minutes—decreases fibrinogen levels and the risk of coronary heart disease.

Diabetes. There is an interrelationship between diabetes and cardiovascular risk factors. In particular, adult-onset diabetes, or Type II diabetes, is associated with obesity and with fat deposits in the abdominal area independent of obesity. People with Type II diabetes have high blood sugar levels, and their bodies are resistant to the hormone insulin. The rate of coronary artery disease is higher in patients with diabetes, and it is not clear whether this is an independent relationship or a consequence of abnormal glucose, lipid, and insulin levels. Whatever the relationship, diet and physical activity provide a "cure" and a return of insulin activity. Weight reduction, increased exercise, and diets high in complex carbohydrates and dietary fiber are all recommended for controlling Type II diabetes. Exercising for 20–30 minutes three times per week, while maintaining a heart rate of 120–140 beats per minute, is recommended (Helmrich et al. 1991).

Table 8–2 summarizes the risk factors associated with cardiovascular disease.

Osteoporosis

The bones that make up the skeleton are constantly being removed by cells called *osteoclasts* and replaced by cells called *osteoblasts.* This removal process is called *resorption* and the replacement is called *formation.* Formation and resorption processes are normally coupled, with bone formation precisely equaling bone resorption to keep the amount of bone constant.

Table 8–2. Risk factors for cardiovascular disease

Family history of cardiovascular disease	High blood pressure
Personal history of premature heart or vascular disease	Excess alcohol intake (i.e., average daily intake of 5–8 drinks)
Elevated cholesterol	Cigarette smoking
Elevated triglycerides	Diabetes
Overweight: waist/hip ratio > 0.85	High fibrinogen levels

Menopause induces an increase in bone *turnover,* or remodeling. This increase peaks 1–2 years after the final menstrual period. Bone is lost more rapidly as resorption increases relative to formation, and calcium is lost from the body. Increasing age also causes an increase in osteoclast activity and a decline in bone mass.

Bone turnover is much more active in what is known as *trabecular,* or "spongy," bone. The bone lost in early postmenopausal bone loss is predominantly of this type, rather than the *cortical,* or "compact," type. The bones of the spine (vertebrae) are predominantly composed of spongy bone, and microfractures of these can be a problem in postmenopausal and elderly women. The thinning of the vertebrae and these fractures can cause compression of the spine and lead to the development of what is sometimes called *dowager's hump* (Figure 8–1) and of pain and disability.

Other clinically important sites of osteoporosis are the wrist and the hip. Hip fractures, which occur predominantly in the elderly female population, are associated with a reduced quality of life and an increased risk of death. Low bone mass is not always the primary reason for hip fracture; the most important cause is falls. Strategies to prevent falls are just as important in the elderly female population as strategies to reduce bone loss. Figure 8–2 is a diagram of the hip joint and bones of the thigh; the area most likely to fracture is the femoral neck.

The decline in estrogen secretion that occurs at menopause is the dominant factor affecting bone metabolism in midlife women. At any point in time, bone mass, which is measured as bone mineral

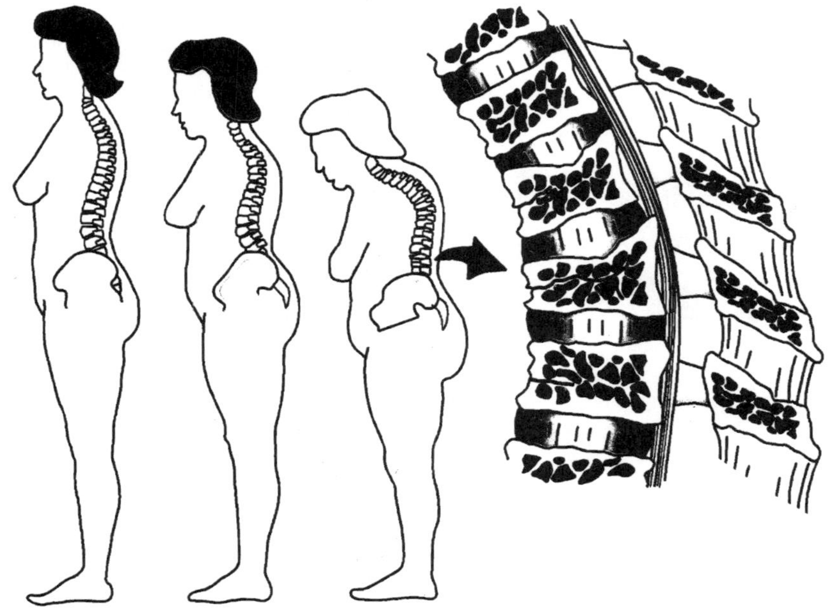

Figure 8–1. Small fractures in the vertebrae cause compression of the spine and the development of so-called dowager's hump.
Source. Australian Dairy Corporation: *Understanding Osteoporosis: A Guide to Prevention and Management.* Melbourne, Australian Dairy Corporation, October 1993. Used with permission.

density, depends on the peak bone mass that has been attained and the amount of bone that has subsequently been lost. The determinants of each of these are discussed in the following pages.

The peak bone mass that has been attained by late adolescence is determined by genetic, nutritional, mechanical, and endocrine (hormone) factors. Approximately 70% of bone mass is determined by genetic factors. White and Asian women are more likely to develop osteoporosis than are black women. Small, lightly built women are also at greater risk. Adequate intake of energy and calcium is necessary, as is mechanical stress being placed on the developing bones. Long periods of immobility cause bone loss. A number of hormones affect the skeleton, and, as already mentioned, estrogen is important in acting directly on bone formation.

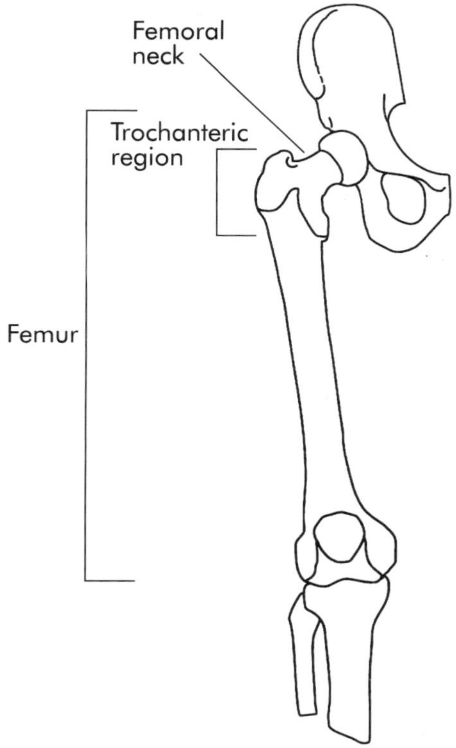

Figure 8–2. The hip joint. The femoral neck is a common site of fracture in elderly persons.

Failure of menstrual cycles (amenorrhea) can adversely affect bone mass and is a particular worry when it occurs in young women. Women who have had a premature menopause, either naturally or because of surgical removal of their ovaries, are at increased risk of developing osteoporosis.

Subsequent bone loss occurs as a result of menopause and aging. Insufficient dietary calcium, excessive intake of caffeine and salt, smoking, and lack of physical exercise are all lifestyle factors that adversely affect bone mass. Other factors known to accelerate bone loss include the use of cortisone-like drugs over a long period.

Bone mineral density can be measured by a number of methods. Dual-energy X-ray absorptiometry (DXA) is the most recent development and is the method of choice for bone densitometry.

It has a high level of precision and subjects the patient to low radiation exposure—approximately 1⁄10 that of a chest X ray. Bone density measurements have a role in clinical practice; for midlife women, it can help in making a decision about whether to start HRT or to assess a woman's response to HRT or to other therapies in preventing osteoporosis.

Calcium and Bone Health

Measures to prevent osteoporosis are aimed at reducing the loss of bone due to menopause and aging. A growing number of controlled trials show that increasing the intake of calcium slows bone loss in postmenopausal women. One study of 122 postmenopausal women in New Zealand showed that increasing the dietary calcium intake from 750 mg to 1,750 mg per day reduced the rate of total body calcium loss by 43% over 2 years (Reid et al. 1993). Researchers have calculated that if a 50% reduction in the rate of bone loss can be achieved from the age of 50 years, the predicted lifetime risk of fracture falls from 17.2% to 6.6%.

Calcium supplementation may be more effective in preventing late rather than early postmenopausal bone loss. This is because, as mentioned previously, the decline in estrogen secretion that occurs around the time of the final menstrual period is the dominant factor affecting bone metabolism. Calcium supplementation may reduce this decline but not override it.

A derivative of vitamin D is required for the normal absorption of calcium from the small intestine. For this reason, adequate vitamin D is required to ensure the positive effect of calcium supplementation on bone mass. Vitamin D is produced mainly through synthesis by the skin, which occurs in the presence of sunlight. Vitamin D deficiency could be a problem in elderly populations of nursing home patients who have been deprived of sunlight. There is no information to date about the effect that the successful anticancer campaign to reduce sun exposure and prevent skin cancer may have on the vitamin D status of the population.

In the controlled trials mentioned above, the average calcium intake was 500–1,000 mg per day, which was then increased by at least 1,000 mg per day. The recommended intake to reduce bone loss is 1,500–2,000 mg per day. This is consistent with other evidence suggesting that to achieve calcium balance in postmenopausal women, an intake of 1,500 mg per day is required (Prince 1993). Calcium balance means that the intake of calcium matches the amount needed by the body and the amount lost from the body—that is, the amount needed to achieve a state of physiological equilibrium. In a study of 16 trials on the effects of physical activity on bone mineral density (Specher 1996), it was reported that physical activity had beneficial effects on bone mineral density at high calcium intakes, with no effect at mean calcium intakes of less than 1,000 mg per day.

Dairy products provide the best dietary source of calcium. The calcium in milk is more easily absorbed by the body than is calcium from any other food source. Low-fat milk and yogurt products provide little or no fat and relatively few calories and are excellent sources of protein, calcium, and certain B vitamins. The calcium content of various foods is listed in Table 8–3. Sardines, salmon, and shellfish are also good sources of calcium.

A high intake of dietary fiber has been shown to reduce calcium absorption, and a high intake of salt increases calcium excretion in urine and sweat. Caffeine has also been shown to have a detrimental effect on bone; recently, several investigators reported that the consumption of caffeine is associated with low bone density and

TABLE 8–3. Food servings providing 300 mg of calcium

35 g (1.2 ounce) cheddar cheese
100 g (3.5 ounces) canned sardines/ salmon with bones
250 ml (8.5 fluid ounces) regular milk
6 oranges
200 g (approximately 1 cup) yogurt
1 kg (2.2 lb) broccoli
135 g (approximately 4 ¾ ounces) ricotta cheese
20 slices of whole-grain bread

osteoporotic fractures (Hernandez-Avila et al. 1993). Caffeine increases the urinary excretion of calcium and could promote a negative calcium balance when ingestion and absorption of calcium are low.

In the Melbourne Women's Midlife Health Project (Dennerstein et al. 1994), 56% of women age 45–55 were found to have a calcium intake of less than 800 mg per day, which is the recommended daily intake for premenopausal women. Half of this group had intakes below 400 mg per day (J. R. Guthrie, unpublished data, 1997).

Physical Activity and Bone Health

Weight-bearing exercise creates a positive stress on bones and helps to increase peak bone mass in younger people and to maintain bone mass in older adults. Recommended weight-bearing activities include walking, jogging, tennis, dancing, and aerobic exercise classes and should be performed regularly.

In one U.S. study (Grove and Londeree 1992), a group of sedentary early postmenopausal women were recruited into an exercise program requiring 60 minutes of organized physical activity three times per week, including 20 minutes of high- or low-impact exercises. (Examples of low-impact activities are fast walking and dancing the Charleston; high-impact activities include running on the spot and knee-to-elbow jumps.) After 1 year, there was no change in the bone mineral density of the lumbar spine of the exercising group, whereas in a matched sedentary control group there was a 6% decline in spinal bone mineral density. The results showed that either low- or high-impact exercise prevented the decline in bone mineral density that occurred in the control group (Grove and Londeree 1992).

In another study (Caplan et al. 1993), a group of postmenopausal women with a mean age of 66 years, participated in a twice-weekly, 60-minute exercise program, including 25 minutes of low-impact aerobic exercise, and worked out at least one other time during the week. After 2 years, the mean percentage change in the bone mineral density of the lumbar spine was a decrease of 0.8% in the exercisers and a decrease of 3.8% in a matched, nonexercising control group. The mean percentage change in the bone mineral content of the trochanter (the top of the shaft of the femur, or thigh bone) was an increase of 9.6% in the exercisers and a decrease of 4.4% in control subjects.

Non–weight-bearing activities, such as swimming and bicycling, have not been considered effective in decreasing bone loss in postmenopausal women. This is true in relation to swimming, but one study (Bloomfield et al. 1993) showed an increase in bone density of the lumbar spine in women who exercised regularly at moderate intensities for 8 months on stationary bicycles. The bone density of the lumbar spine in sedentary control subjects was shown to have decreased during this time. No significant differences were found in the change in bone density of the femoral neck of the cyclists and the control subjects.

Both physical activity and calcium intake are extremely important in the maintenance of bone health at the time of menopause and as women age. These are the two most important factors within human control that can affect the bone degeneration that occurs gradually in all humans. A program of increased physical activity and increased calcium intake is attractive because it is relatively easy to implement and there are no unwanted side effects, provided that the exercise program is not initially too strenuous. Also, recent evidence shows that high calcium intake is not associated with the formation of kidney stones (Curhan et al. 1993).

Estrogen therapy does prevent bone loss in postmenopausal women, but recent research has determined that at least 10 years of estrogen therapy after menopause are necessary for a long-term protective effect on bone mineral density. Even therapy for this length of time may be insufficient to protect women age 75 years and older from fracture (Lindsay 1993).

Genitourinary Problems

Estrogen deficiency leads to tissue changes in the genital tract and bladder, resulting in alterations in sexual function and urinary problems. Exercise does not provide a "cure" for the former, although an active sex life is one form of physical activity and sensitive love-making will help. A number of nonhormonal vaginal lubricants are available.

Urinary problems, such as stress incontinence, can be helped by exercises to strengthen the muscles of the pelvic floor. The pelvic floor muscles support the bladder, uterus, and bowel and are not strengthened by the forms of leisure-time physical activity referred to in relation to cardiovascular and osteoporotic problems.

To strengthen your pelvic floor muscles, first make yourself aware of what it feels like to contract them. These muscles can be tested by starting the flow of urine and then stopping it. Once you have become aware of these muscle contractions, practice them. Do three pelvic floor contractions regularly during the day, for example, when you shower or brush your teeth. Do not stop and start the urine flow as an exercise, only as a test to identify the proper muscles. Starting and stopping the flow of urine on a regular basis can result in urinary problems.

More information on pelvic floor muscles and urinary problems is beyond the scope of this chapter. An excellent book on the topic is *Women's Waterworks: Curing Incontinence,* by Pauline E. Chiarelli (1989).

Hot Flashes

In the Melbourne Women's Midlife Health Project, the level of physical activity (measured by duration and intensity) had no significant effect on women's experiences of the frequency and intensity of hot flashes. However, exercising at least once a week was associated with lower levels of overall health-related complaints (Morse et al. 1994) and better well-being (Dennerstein et al. 1994).

No exercise prescription will alleviate hot flashes. However, the benefits of physical activity for all the other reasons mentioned should make exercise a mandatory part of a woman's lifestyle. In addition, women who have exercised strenuously are familiar with feelings of increased skin temperature and sweating (the mechanisms used to cool the body due to heat produced during muscular activity), so the feelings associated with a hot flash are not foreign or necessarily uncomfortable.

Phytoestrogens

Some plants contain plant estrogens (phytoestrogens), substances that mimic the actions of estrogens. They are generally considered to be extremely weak compared with human hormones, but, when taken in high enough concentrations in the diet, they can alleviate menopausal symptoms. Table 8–4 lists plants and foods known to contain reasonable levels of phytoestrogens. Legumes display estrogenic activity, particularly soy products, such as soybeans, soy flour, soy grits, tofu, and bean curd. The soy protein content of 1 ounce (28 g) of soy flour is 10–13 g, of 8 ounces (226 g) of soy milk is 4–10 g, and of 4 ounces (113 g) of tofu is 8–13 g (Dwyer et al. 1994).

The variation in the incidence of hot flashes among women of different ethnic backgrounds may be due in part to a variation in the consumption of soy products. Japanese women, for example, have a much higher intake of soy products and a lower incidence of reporting of hot flashes than Australian women. Australian studies have shown that in postmenopausal women, additional soy flour and linseed can improve the vaginal mucosa, and additional soy flour can assist in relieving hot flashes (Murkies et al. 1995; Wilcox et al. 1991). Further research is necessary to elucidate the levels of phytoestrogens that may help relieve menopausal symp-

Table 8–4. Phytoestrogen-containing plants, foods, and herbs

Alfalfa	Clover	Hops	Soybeans
Aniseed	Common beans	Licorice	Viburnum
Avena	Corn	Parsley	Wheat bran and wheat germ
Basil	Dill	Peas	
Cabbage	Fennel	Rice bran	
Caraway	Garlic	Sage	
Chervil	Ginseng	Senecio	

toms and whether there may be any untoward effects of phytoestrogens on health.

What Are the Physical Activities of Midlife Women?

Because in this chapter I emphasize the need for physical activity, it is interesting to look at women's participation in leisure-time physical activities, in terms of type and duration, from ages 45 to 55. In the Melbourne Women's Midlife Health Project, it was found that the most popular activities were walking and gardening; 83% of women walked for pleasure, and 77% cultivated their gardens. Other popular activities were swimming, home exercises, and dancing. There was low participation in more strenuous physical activities, such as aerobics, squash playing, and jogging (Guthrie et al. 1995).

Only 10% of the above population had very low levels of exercise—that is, less than an hour per week. In total, about one-third of the women exercised less than 3 hours per week. If weekly exercise energy expenditure is considered—that is, the intensity of the activities as well as the length of time they are performed—one-third of the total cohort were below the level considered optimal for protection against coronary artery disease. Although there have been population studies of midlife women in other countries, those published to date have not provided details about the types of physical activities in which the women participated.

Menopause is often associated with a decrease in physical fitness. This is not related to the hormonal changes of the menopause but probably reflects a loss of functional capacity due to a natural age-related deterioration and a decrease in physical activity. It has been shown that the ability to improve cardiorespiratory fitness is independent of menopausal status. In a U.S. study (Cowan and Gregory 1985), two groups of women, one premenopausal and the other postmenopausal, exercised 4 days a week for 9 weeks at an intensity of 80% of their age-adjusted maximum heart rate (maxi-

Table 8–5. Health checklist

Eat more fruits and vegetables
Eat less fat, especially less animal fat
Be physically active
Avoid being overweight
Drink alcohol in moderation, if at all

mum heart rate = 220 minus age). The duration of the exercise was gradually increased from 17 to 44 minutes. The cardiovascular fitness of these women was significantly improved over that of two nonexercising control groups. There was no effect of menopause on any of the measures of cardiovascular endurance (Cowan and Gregory 1985).

In summary, the benefits of regular physical activity are that it improves blood lipid profiles, reduces blood pressure, reduces weight, maintains bone density, and improves coordination and muscle strength, and hence reduces the risk of falling. Table 8–5 summarizes five important health recommendations.

Exercise is not a panacea. However, together with appropriate lifestyle and nutritional measures, it can be considered a useful additive to, and in many instances an alternative to, hormone therapy.

References

Bloomfield SA, Williams NI, Lamb DR, et al: Non-weight-bearing exercise may increase lumbar spine bone mineral density in healthy postmenopausal women. American Journal of Physical Medicine and Rehabilitation 72:204–208, 1993

Caplan GA, Ward JA, Lord SR: The benefits of exercise in postmenopausal women. Australian Journal of Public Health 17:23–26, 1993

Cauley JA, La Porte RE, Sandler RB, et al: The relationship of physical activity to high density lipoprotein cholesterol in postmenopausal women. Journal of Chronic Diseases 39:687–697, 1986

Chiarelli PE: Women's Waterworks: Curing Incontinence. Sydney, Australia, Century Magazines, 1989

Cowan MM, Gregory LW: Responses of pre- and post-menopausal females to aerobic conditioning. Medicine and Science in Sports and Exercise 17:138–142, 1985

Curhan GC, Willett WC, Rimm EB, et al: A prospective study of dietary calcium and other nutrients and the risk of symptomatic kidney stones. New England Journal of Medicine 328:833–838, 1993

Dennerstein L, Smith AMA, Morse C: Psychological well-being, mid-life and the menopause. Maturitas 20:1–11, 1994

Dwyer JT, Goldin BR, Saul N, et al: Tofu and soy drinks contain phytoestrogens. Journal of the American Dietetic Association 94(7):739–743, 1994

Ernst E: Regular exercise reduces fibrinogen levels: a review of longitudinal studies. British Journal of Sports Medicine 27(3):175–176, 1993

Grove KA, Londeree BR: Bone density in postmenopausal women: high impact vs low impact exercise. Medicine and Science in Sports and Exercise 24(11):1190–1194, 1992

Guthrie JR, Smith AA, Dennerstein L, et al: Physical activity and the menopause experience. Maturitas 20:71–80, 1995

Helmrich SP, Ragland DR, Leung RW, et al: Physical activity and reduced occurrence of non-insulin dependent diabetes. New England Journal of Medicine 325:147–152, 1991

Hernandez-Avila M, Stampfer MJ, Ravnikar VA, et al: Caffeine and other predictors of bone density among pre- and perimenopausal women. Epidemiology 4:128–134, 1993

Lindsay R: Hormone replacement therapy for the prevention and treatment of osteoporosis. American Journal of Medicine 95 (suppl 5a):37–39, 1993

Morse C, Smith AA, Dennerstein L, et al: The treatment-seeking woman at menopause. Maturitas 18:161–173, 1994

Murkies AL, Lombard C, Strauss BJG, et al: Dietary flour supplementation decreases postmenopausal hot flushes: effect of soy and wheat. Maturitas 21:189–195, 1995

Notelovitz M: Exercise and health maintenance in menopausal women. Annals of the New York Academy of Sciences 592:204–220, 1990

Owens JF, Matthews KA, Wing RR, et al: Can physical activity mitigate the effects of aging in middle-aged women? Circulation 85:1265–1270, 1992

Prince R: The calcium controversy revisited: implications of new data. Medical Journal of Australia 159:404–407, 1993

Reaven PD, Barrett-Connor E, Edelstein S: Relation between leisure-time physical activity and blood pressure in older women. Circulation 83:559–565, 1991

Reid IR, Ames RN, Evans MC, et al: Effect of calcium supplementation on bone loss in postmenopausal women. New England Journal of Medicine 328:460–464, 1993
Specher BL: Evidence for an interaction between calcium intake and physical activity on changes in bone mineral density. Journal of Bone and Mineral Research 11:1539–1544, 1996
Wilcox G, Wahlqvist ML, Burger HG, et al: Oestrogenic effects of plant foods on postmenopausal women. British Medical Journal 301:905–906, 1991
Wing RR, Matthews KA, Kuller LH, et al: Weight gain at the time of the menopause. Archives of Internal Medicine 151:97–102, 1991

CHAPTER 9

What Do Natural Therapies Have to Offer the Debate?

Assunta Hunter

The term *natural therapies* is an umbrella term that encompasses a range of disciplines, including nutrition, herbal medicine, homeopathy, traditional Chinese medicine, and acupuncture. These forms of medicine are often loosely called "alternative" or "complementary" medicines in industrialized societies. In fact, however, many of them, such as acupuncture and Chinese herbal medicine, are based on the traditional medicine systems of Europe and Asia. All of these disciplines share an underlying belief in the body's ability to return to some kind of equilibrium, given the appropriate support.

Natural therapies regard treatment as nutritive and ultimately restorative of normal physiological processes. Their methods and medicines are generally guided by the Hippocratic principle—"First, do no harm"—and include the use of food therapies and nutritional supplements; herbal and homeopathic remedies; and noningestive therapies, such as massage, manipulation, and acupuncture (Newman Turner 1984).

The basic philosophical tenet of these therapies is the promotion of health rather than the treatment of the symptoms of disease. The emphasis in practice is on influencing the body's recuperative functions rather than treating only symptoms or pathologies. Treatment is very much based on the individual. Similar symptoms arising in different patients are often treated in different ways. The basis for this approach is to treat underlying weaknesses, which may be quite different in different people. For this reason, there is no set herbal formula or any one treatment that can be used for every patient as treatment for menopausal symptoms.

"Natural" Remedies

The term *natural* is often equated with safe and nontoxic. However, there are a small proportion of herbal remedies that can be toxic, especially in untrained hands. In general, it can be said that herbal medicines and natural products (e.g., vitamin and mineral supplements and food supplements) have very low toxic potentials. But it should be emphasized that, if these substances are being used as medicines, they should be prescribed by a practitioner who has specialized knowledge of their actions and side effects. Like all therapeutic regimens, natural therapies must be treated with respect and supervised by someone who has expertise in the area and the patient's welfare in mind.

It is difficult to compare natural products with conventional pharmaceutical products, which are generally single constituents that are standardized, purified, and dispensed in exact quantities. Although natural products in most industrialized nations are subjected to manufacturing standards, most herbs and many food supplements contain a variety of active ingredients and a complex array of substances found in unrefined raw materials. The concern is often expressed that, because of this, these substances may be difficult to prescribe safely. However, whole plant products often contain a unique balance of constituents that actually diminish the risk of side effects and protect against toxicity. For example, willow bark (from which aspirin is derived) has anti-inflammatory and fever-reducing actions that are similar to those of aspirin, but, because of the balance of its other constituents, the whole plant does not cause stomach irritation or gastric bleeding.

The therapeutic index of most natural products is very wide and the potential for toxicity very small. Many of the difficulties associated with natural products can be ascribed to inappropriate self-medication, poor labeling, and governmental unwillingness to regulate the profession or to set the same safety standards of manufacture.

Natural therapies offer an alternative to hormone replacement therapy (HRT). It is oversimplifying the matter considerably to ask only whether or not to take HRT . In reality, there are many other options, including the use of natural therapies for the treatment of any symptoms that occur, as well as for the maintenance of good health.

For women embarking on treatment in menopause, natural therapies have the advantage of focusing broadly on improving general health while posing minimal risks in terms of side effects. When appropriately prescribed, natural therapies can be very effective in the treatment of not just hot flashes but also many other symptoms, such as night sweats, frequent urination, vaginal dryness, and emotional lability. Using natural therapies in menopause can be appropriate for women in whom the use of HRT is contraindicated. These therapies are also used by women who have found HRT to be ineffective for their symptoms or to create unwanted side effects. And of course, a large proportion of women using natural therapies do so because they prefer this style of medicine.

Of these women, it may well be said that they have a strong belief in, and desire to use, nonpharmaceutical drugs. Even in the face of severe menopausal symptoms, they prefer a strict dietary regimen and herbal or homeopathic and vitamin therapies as their medicines. And although it may require learning how to reduce their stress levels and how to strengthen their bones with exercise, this is what they prefer.

Menopause is seen by natural therapists as a part of the cyclic nature of women's hormonal lives rather than as a state of estrogen deficiency. The aim of natural therapies at this time is to ease the woman through this transitional phase by maintaining her in the best possible health on all levels—physical, emotional, and spiritual. Treatment therefore encompasses all these levels of care.

On the physical level, treatment may include dietary advice (and possibly also supplementation), herbal and/or homeopathic treatment, and advice about exercise and lifestyle. In this chapter, I focus largely on the nutritional and herbal approaches to the treatment of menopausal symptoms.

A variety of scientifically based information supports the use of natural treatment strategies. Historically, traditional medicines have been empirically based; their treatments have been developed through experience passed down through the generations. In the last three to four decades, there has been much scientific research in the areas of nutrition and herbal medicine that validates, from a scientific viewpoint, some of these forms of treatment (Beckham 1995a, 1995b; Bone 1995; Markiewicz et al. 1993). Clinical research is still incomplete, and natural therapists use a combination of scientifically based information and empirically based tradition as a basis for practice. Much of the useful research in these areas comes from the disciplines of plant chemistry (phytochemistry), plant therapy (phytotherapy), cross-cultural comparisons of dietary patterns and disease incidence (Adlercreutz 1990; Adlercreutz et al. 1986, 1992a; Miksicek 1993; Wilcox et al. 1990), and clinical nutrition (Chapuy et al. 1992; Prince 1993; Prince et al. 1991; Reid et al. 1993).

Natural Therapies

Decreased production of estrogens and progesterone by the ovaries is a major aspect of the processes of menopause. Natural therapy's approach to treatment is to improve the body's physiological adaption to this process in a number of ways. There are both direct and indirect strategies for supporting this adaption.

Treatments Directly Affecting Hormone Levels

One group of treatments are often loosely described as having a phytoestrogenic action. More specifically, they can be classified as using the following:

Herbs and foods that supply phytoestrogenic substances

Herbs and foods that are metabolized into phytoestrogenic substances in the gut

Herbs that affect the symptoms of menopause by acting on pituitary hormones

Treatments Indirectly Supporting the Body's Adaptive Responses

Certain herbal and nutritional strategies affect hormone levels indirectly and are part of a broadly based, natural-therapy approach to the treatment of menopausal symptoms. These treatments are characterized by the following:

- Using herbs to support the body's use of adrenally produced estrones
- Encouraging the use of estrones supplied by fat metabolism
- Ensuring the availability of the nutritional building blocks necessary for the internal production and activity of estrogen
- Ensuring optimal supply and absorption of calcium and magnesium in the diet

Strategies Directly Affecting Hormone Levels

A variety of ways are used in natural therapies to augment the body's production of estrogen to treat menopausal symptoms. Whereas orthodox medicine has supplied synthetic or semisynthetic estrogens to bolster the falling levels of estrogens produced by the ovaries, herbal medicine in particular has used plant-derived medicines that either act like estrogens within the body or cause the estrogens produced by the body to work for longer periods of time. A broad general division may be made between herbs containing chemical substances known as *steroidal saponins* and substances called *phytoestrogens* (literally, "plant estrogens"). Phytoestrogens are also described in Chapter 8.

Plants such as licorice (*Glycyrrhiza glabra*) and Mexican yam (*Dioscorea villosa*), which contain steroidal saponins, have a close structural relationship to the hormones that are produced internally by the body. Historically, the Mexican yam was used as the source of chemicals to produce the first contraceptive pills. Licorice has long been used in menopausal treatment because of its ability to support the adrenal glands. Licorice enables the hormones produced by these glands to continue to work for longer periods (Tamura et al. 1979).

Another saponin-containing plant is black cohosh (*Cimicifuga racemosa*). This plant has a long tradition of empirical use and has also been subject to extensive chemical research and clinical trials, particularly in Germany (Stellang 1994). It is particularly effective in reducing hot flashes, and there is evidence of its ability to positively alter the turnover in vaginal cells, thus reducing the symptoms of vaginal dryness (Stoll 1987; Warneke 1985). It is used extensively in Europe for the treatment of menopausal symptoms.

The significance of plants with estrogenic activity lies in their ability to act like estrogens within the body. At menopause, the body's internal production of estrogen is low, and many estrogen receptors are vacant. In this situation, herbs and foods that occupy these receptor sites have an estrogenic effect and consequently have a positive effect in reducing menopausal symptoms such as flushing, vaginal dryness, and night sweats. It has been suggested that the high levels of particular isoflavones in the diet of Japanese women—due to the widespread use of soybeans and soy products in a traditional Japanese diet—may be part of the explanation for the infrequency of hot flashes and other menopausal symptoms in the Japanese population (Adlercreutz et al. 1992b).

Plants containing phytoestrogens belong to two main chemical groupings, the isoflavones and the lignans. Both of these kinds of plant estrogens are widely distributed in the foodstuffs of a normal diet. The group known as isoflavones contains a large number of well-known foods, including soybeans (and other soy products, such as tofu, tempeh, miso, and soybean shoots), chickpeas, mung beans, alfalfa, rice, and whole grains. The lignans are also widely distributed in the foodstuffs of a Western diet. They are found in linseeds, sunflower seeds, sesame seeds, soybeans, buckwheat, and millet, to name a few. Herbs that are used medicinally for their phytoestrogenic activity include the following:

Red clover (*Trifolium praetense*)
Hops (*Humulus lupulus*)
Oatstraw (*Avena sativa*)
St. John's wort (*Hypericum perforatum*)

Treatments Indirectly Supporting the Body's Adaptive Responses in Menopause

In keeping with the general approach to treating the individual and supporting normal physiological processes, natural therapies use a number of strategies that may be loosely called "adaptive." These are primarily ways of encouraging the adaptive processes that are part of the normal bodily response to lower levels of estrogens.

As part of the menopausal transition, there is increased reliance on adrenally produced estrones. Natural therapies use a number of herbs (often referred to as "adaptogens") to extend the activity of adrenal hormones in the body. These herbs are described as improving the body's response to stress in a number of ways (Wagner et al. 1994). Herbs such as licorice, Siberian ginseng, and Korean ginseng fall into this category.

Another feature of the metabolic changes that take place in menopause is the increased use of estrones supplied by fat metabolism. This metabolic pathway is active only when there is a body fat level of at least 20%. Knowing this, however, can be useful to women as part of their overall dietary reorientation at menopause.

It is also important to ensure that all the nutritional building blocks necessary for the production of estrogen internally and for its optimal activity are available. Clinical studies have demonstrated the usefulness of vitamin E in reducing the severity of hot flashes and other symptoms associated with menopause, such as dry skin and irritable mucous membranes (Werbach 1989). Chinese angelica (dong quai), rather than containing plant estrogens, as is sometimes claimed, seems to be effective in reducing menopausal symptoms by extending the action of the body's own estrogen through its antioxidant and vitamin E-enhancing effects (Bensky and Gamble 1986).

Ensuring an optimal supply of both calcium and magnesium in the diet and encouraging their intestinal absorption and utilization are other important aspects of indirect support to the body's normal adaptive responses. Both of these minerals are vital to the continuing strength of the bones (as are a number of other minerals, such as phosphorus, zinc, boron, and silicon). Magnesium supplementation at appropriate levels may be as important as calcium in maintaining bone strength. Individuals with osteoporosis have been shown to have unusually low levels of magnesium in their bone matrix (Werbach 1989).

Natural therapy's approach to the treatment of menopausal symptoms is thus both direct and indirect. It not only supplies plant estrogens but also encourages the body's transition to other sources of estrogens that can be produced postmenopausally. Rather than simply supplying estrogen, natural therapy focuses on encouraging the hormone's optimal assimilation and utilization by a number of physiological processes. It attempts to support normal processes and to reduce symptoms by ensuring the body's supply of nutritional building blocks for this process.

The management of menopause with natural therapies is an option that an increasing number of women are choosing. Although there is ample evidence to substantiate many of the strategies developed by natural therapies, there is also a need for continued clinical research by natural therapists in this area.

References

Adlercreutz H: Western diet and Western diseases: some hormonal and biochemical mechanisms and associations. Scandinavian Journal of Clinical and Laboratory Investigation 50(suppl 201):3–23, 1990

Adlercreutz H, Fotsis T, Bannwort K, et al: Determination of urinary lignans and phytoestrogen metabolites, potential antiestrogens and anticarcinogens: urine of women on various habitual diets. Journal of Steroid Biochemistry 25(5B):791–797, 1986

Adlercreutz H, Mousavi Y, Clark J, et al: Dietary phytoestrogens and cancer: in vitro and in vivo studies. Journal of Steroid Biochemistry and Molecular Biology 41:331–337, 1992a

Adlercreutz H, Hamalainen E, Gorbach S, et al: Dietary phyto-oestrogens and the menopause in Japan (letter). Lancet 339:1233, 1992b

Beckham N: Menopause: A Positive Approach Using Natural Therapies. Sydney, Viking/Penguin, 1995a

Beckham N: Phytoestrogens and compounds that affect oestrogen metabolism: Part 1. Australian Journal of Medical Herbalism 7(1):11–16, 1995b (Note: the bibliography for this article is contained in Beckham N: Phytoestrogens and compounds that affect oestrogen metabolism: part 2. Australian Journal of Medical Herbalism 7(2):27–33, 1995)

Bensky D, Gamble A: Chinese Herbal Medicine Materia Medica. Seattle, WA, Eastland Press, 1986

Bone K: Oestrogen modulation. The Modern Phytotherapist 1(2):8–10, 1995

Chapuy MC, Arlot ME, Duboeuf F, et al: Vitamin D3 and calcium to prevent hip fractures in elderly women. New England Journal of Medicine 327:1637–1642, 1992

Markiewicz L, Garey J, Adlercreutz H, et al: In vitro bioassays of nonsteroidal phytoestrogens. Journal of Steroid Biochemistry and Molecular Biology 45(5):399–405, 1993

Miksicek RJ: Commonly occurring plant flavinoids have oestrogenic activity. Molecular Pharmacology 44:37–43, 1993

Newman Turner R: Naturopathic Medicine: Treating the Whole Person. Wellingborough, Northamptonshire, UK, Thorsons, 1984

Prince R: The calcium controversy revisited: implications of new data. Medical Journal of Australia 159:404–407, 1993

Prince RI, Smith M, Dick IM, et al: Prevention of post-menopausal osteoporosis. New England Journal of Medicine 325:1189–1195, 1991

Reid IR, Ames RW, Evans MC, et al: The effect of calcium supplementation on bone loss in post-menopausal women. New England Journal of Medicine 328:460–464, 1993

Stellang K: Cimicifuga racemosa. Canadian Journal of Herbalism, April 1994, pp 20–25

Stoll W: Phytopharmacin influences atrophic vaginal epithelium: double blind study—cimicifuga vs estrogenic substances (translation). Therapeutikan 1:23–32, 1987

Tamura Y, Nishikawa T, Yamada K: Effects of glycyrrhetinic acid and its derivatives on delta-4,5-alpha- and 5-beta-reductase in rat liver. Arzneimittelforschung 29:647–649, 1979
Wagner H, Norr H, Winterhoff H: Plant adaptogens. Phytomedicine 1:63–76, 1994
Warneke G: Influencing menopausal symptoms with a phytotherapeutic agent. Reprint from De Mediziniche Welt 36:871–874, 1985
Werbach MR: Nutritional Influences on Illness. London, Thorsons, 1989, pp 331–341
Wilcox G, Wahlqvist ML, Burger HG, et al: Oestrogenic effects of plant foods in post menopausal women. Br J Med 301:905–906, 1990

CHAPTER 10

Summary: What World Health Organization Experts Say

Lorraine Dennerstein

In June 1994 the World Health Organization (WHO) convened a meeting of the Scientific Group on Research on the Menopause in the 1990s. Gathered together in Geneva were 30 international experts from a wide range of disciplines: gynecology, endocrinology, oncology, general practice, demography, psychiatry, anthropology, statistics, epidemiology, women's health, bone metabolism, gerontology, and internal medicine. A wide range of countries and continents were also represented, including Australia, Asia (China, Indonesia, Thailand, and Japan), Africa (Kenya, Uganda, and Nigeria), Western Europe (the United Kingdom), Eastern Europe (Hungary), the Middle East (Egypt), Scandinavia (Finland and Denmark), South America (Brazil), and North America. Below is a summary of the discussions that took place at the meeting. A full report was published in 1996 by the WHO Technical Report Series (WHO Scientific Group 1996).

What Is Menopause?

The experts agreed that menopause is a normal physiological event that occurs in all women who live to middle age. They also noted that a woman's health status at menopause is only one point in a continuum of life phases and is largely determined by prior health status, reproductive pattern, lifestyle, and environmental exposures.

Menopause Around the World

It is estimated that there are more than 470 million women worldwide age 50 years and over. Women's age at menopause may be somewhat younger for women in developing countries. The life expectancy for women who reach 50 years of age is fairly similar worldwide, varying from 27 to 32 years for most countries. In 1990, 25 million women worldwide passed through menopause. The number of postmenopausal women is expected to increase sharply over the next 40 years, to 1.2 billion by 2030.

At present, 60% of postmenopausal women live in developing countries. Because population growth rates are much faster in developing countries, this proportion will increase to 76% by 2030. Yet most research has involved women in industrialized countries of Europe and North America.

Findings indicate that menopause may be perceived and experienced very differently in different cultures. Participants from sub-Saharan Africa and Asia reported that menopause may be associated with positive social changes for some women. One problem is that the relatively few studies carried out in developing countries have used similar research methods and have asked the same research questions as studies designed for industrialized countries. Yet these sorts of studies have not considered whether there may be other questions of importance to the health of women in these countries. Nor do they take into account the very different set of factors that have framed the health of women in developing countries. The health and well-being of all women is strongly influenced by the cultural and economic settings in which they live and by their prior life experiences, including the physical demands of their work and home life, environmental exposure, reproductive experiences, dietary adequacy, and the availability of public health and health care services.

Studies that have investigated women's experiences of symptoms during the menopausal transition generally have found fewer symptoms reported by women of cultures other than those of the industrialized world. Further, some studies have reported a different pattern of symptoms. There may also be a lower incidence for longer-term problems, such as osteoporotic fractures. For example, older Mayan women have bone demineralization but a lower incidence of osteoporotic fractures. Even within industrialized countries, there are significant differences for different ethnic groups. White Americans experience significantly more hip fractures than do Mexican Americans or Japanese women living in Hawaii. Rates of coronary heart disease and breast cancer may also be lower among postmenopausal women in Asia, although accurate data are not available for many countries.

Symptoms

The experts noted that symptoms that occur in many women during the menopausal transition are self-limiting and not life-threatening but may be troubling for the women concerned. There are possible delayed effects of the menopause on many organ systems of the body, particularly the cardiovascular and skeletal systems.

Consistently associated with menopause in the industrialized countries have been the vasomotor symptoms of hot flashes and night sweats. These symptoms can be relieved with estrogen or estrogen plus progestin. Nonpharmacological therapies such as behavior therapies have also reduced the frequency of hot flashes.

Vaginal thinning, with resulting painful intercourse, can be alleviated by estrogen therapy. Vaginal lubricants are useful for dyspareunia. Continuing sexual activity helps protect against vaginal thinning. Urinary symptoms, such as urgency, discomfort, and increased frequency, may relate in part to menopausal hormonal changes and may respond to estrogen therapy.

Cardiovascular Diseases

Cardiovascular diseases are the most common causes of death in women and men in almost all parts of the world. The experts reviewed epidemiological studies in which the risk for coronary heart disease was on the order of 50% lower in postmenopausal women treated with oral estrogens than in untreated women. It was noted that there may be possible biases in the studies (see Chapter 5) and that there is a need for large, randomized, controlled trials of hormone replacement therapy (HRT), such as the Women's Health Initiative (Chapter 5).

The results thus far indicate that the protective effect of HRT is greater for women who have had induced surgical menopause, had experienced natural menopause before age 55, were current users of estrogen, and had used long-term estrogen. Because such use is known to increase the risk of endometrial cancer, combined therapy in which a progestin is added is recommended for women who have not undergone hysterectomy. Estrogen use has been shown in a few studies to be associated with less narrowing of the coronary arteries and a higher survival rate for women who had 70% or greater narrowing.

Osteoporosis and Fractures

Osteoporosis and associated fractures are a major cause of mortality and morbidity worldwide, although the prevalence varies among countries and among population groups within countries. Black Americans have greater bone mass than do white Americans, and

Asian Americans have less. Hip fracture rates are highest in the United States and lowest in Africa. Bone density alone does not explain hip fracture rates, because fracture rates are lower in Japan than in the United States, despite similar low bone density in both countries. Women have a consistently higher bone loss with age and a higher fracture risk than men. Both low bone mass and the propensity to falls are contributors to fractures. The propensity to falls is increased by certain drugs and alcohol, lack of exercise, muscle weakness, and chronic illness.

The experts recommended that osteoporosis prevention take place throughout life. Measures include adequate calcium intake, moderate exercise, and avoidance of smoking and excessive alcohol (see Chapter 8 for more details). Because vitamin D levels fall markedly with age, supplementation may be needed for the elderly and has been shown to stop bone loss and reduce vertebral fracture rates.

Hormone therapy with estrogen or estrogen plus progestin was found to maintain bone density in postmenopausal women as long as the hormone therapy continues. Hormone therapy may thus be used for prevention of osteoporosis and is also used to treat established osteoporosis.

Breast Cancer

Breast cancer is the most frequent malignant disease in women in all developed countries except Japan, and the incidence of breast cancer is increasing worldwide. The risk of breast cancer is increased by exposure to endogenous estrogen, as indicated by female sex, early age at menarche, late age at menopause, and obesity in postmenopausal women. Bilateral oophorectomy at an early age reduces the risk of breast cancer. Observational studies have found that the use of estrogen by postmenopausal women for less than 5 years appears to have little or no effect on the risk of breast cancer. Use for 5–9 years may have a small increased risk. Use for 10 years or more may be associated with a 30%–80% increase in risk. The experts found that the addition of progestin or androgen to estrogen may be associated with an increase in the risk of breast cancer. The public health effects of an increased risk of breast cancer from long-term HRT may depend on the underlying risk of breast cancer in the country concerned.

Gynecological Cancers

There was strong evidence that cancer of the endometrium is increased by the use of unopposed estrogen (i.e., without the addition of a progestin). Increased duration of use markedly increases this risk. The addition of progestin to estrogen therapy was found to lower this risk. The current clinical recommendation is that a progestin be added to the HRT regimen for at least 10 days per month when estrogen is prescribed for a woman who has not undergone hysterectomy. The experts found no evidence of any association between HRT and cancer of the ovary, cervix, or vulva.

Hormone Therapies

The WHO experts concluded that the peri- and postmenopausal phases of life are part of the aging process that do not necessarily require therapeutic intervention. Acute symptoms, such as hot flashes and vaginal dryness, may require short-term use of HRT. Existing evidence for accelerated bone loss after menopause, and possibly increased cardiovascular risk, suggests that longer-term pharmacological and nonpharmacological interventions may be appropriate for certain postmenopausal women.

The WHO Scientific Group strongly recommended that all midlife women be encouraged to pursue healthy lifestyles that may include smoking cessation, regular exercise, balanced diet, and safe sex. Such therapy is likely to be most effective when it is part of an overall life plan because lifestyle behaviors such as dietary patterns, regular exercise, and abstention from smoking have far-reaching beneficial effects on health.

Hormone therapies have been recommended to reduce the immediate and long-term consequences of menopause. The goals of therapy must be clearly understood—that is, whether therapy is for short-term relief of symptoms or for longer-term use to reduce risk of cardiovascular disease and fractures. The risks and benefits vary with length of use and the type of hormones used.

At present, the experts could recommend that, for women who have had a hysterectomy and for whom estrogen alone can be prescribed, the benefits of HRT exceed the risks and therapy can be prescribed at a reasonable cost. For women with an intact uterus, progestin should be added to the therapy. The results are then less certain. Women at high risk of coronary heart disease may benefit from such therapy. Those at high risk of breast cancer may have no remaining benefit and may even have a reduction in life expectancy. Early natural or induced menopause before age 40 is an indication for long-term hormone treatment at least up to the usual age of natural menopause. Other disagreeable side effects of hormone therapy, such as irregular bleeding (or even regular bleeding), breast tenderness, premenstrual-type symptoms, the need for regular medication, physician visits, and fear of cancer also have to be considered, as do other possible benefits, such as preservation of urinary and sexual function and improved bone density.

Reference

World Health Organization Scientific Group: Research on the Menopause in the 1990s. WHO Technical Report Series 866. Geneva, World Health Organization, 1996

Index

Page numbers printed in **boldface** type refer to tables or figures.